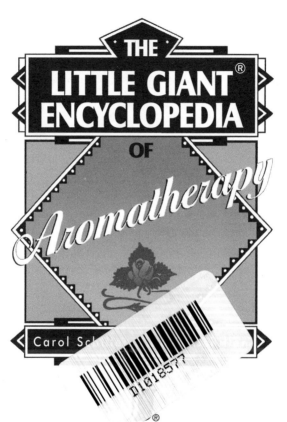

THE
LITTLE GIANT®
ENCYCLOPEDIA

OF

Aromatherapy

Carol Sc...

Sterling Publishing Co., Inc.

Library of Congress Cataloging-in-Publication Data

Schiller, Carol.
  The little giant encyclopedia of aromatherapy / Carol Schiller &
David Schiller.
    p.   cm.
  Includes index.
  ISBN 0–8069–2065–3
  1. Aromatherapy Encyclopedias. I. Schiller, David, 1942–   .
II. Title.
RM666.A68S357 1999
615'.321—dc21   99–33939

10 8 6 4 2 1 3 5 7 9

Published by Sterling Publishing Company, Inc.
387 Park Avenue South, New York, New York 10016
© 1999 by Carol Schiller and David Schiller
Distributed in Canada by Sterling Publishing
c/o Canadian Manda Group, One Atlantic Avenue, Suite 105
Toronto, Ontario, Canada M6K 3E7
Distributed in Great Britain and Europe by Cassell PLC
Wellington House, 125 Strand, London WC2R 0BB, England
Distributed in Australia by Capricorn Link (Australia) Pty Ltd.
P.O. Box 6651, Baulkham Hills, Business Centre, NSW 2153,
Australia
Manufactured in the United States of America
Sterling ISBN 0–8069–2065–3

ACKNOWLEDGMENTS

We would like to thank these people at Sterling Publishing who made this book possible:

Sheila Anne Barry, Acquisitions Manager
John Woodside, Editorial Director
Charles Nurnberg, Executive Vice President

This book is dedicated to people who are enthralled by the extraordinary magnificence of nature— her wonders, her beauty, and her infinite intelligence.

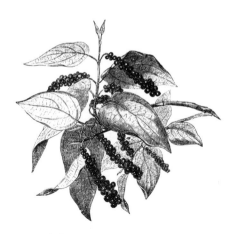

Black Pepper (*Piper nigrum*)

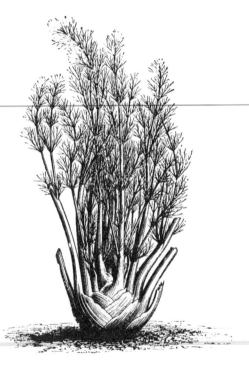

Sweet Fennel (*Foeniculum vulgare*)

Contents

CHAPTER 4

Inhalation for Mood & Effect 169

CHAPTER 6

Home Products

CHAPTER 9

Introduction to Aromatherapy

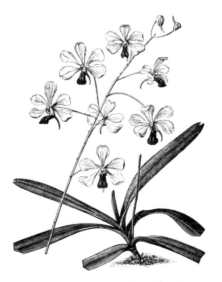

Vanda Orchid (*Vanda caerulescens*)

*A*n appetizing aroma, emitted from food we enjoy, travels into our nasal passages and finds its way to smell receptors. Suddenly, our appetite increases, our mouth waters, digestive juices flow, and our mood lifts. A pleasing scent wafts through the air, dispersing its sublime aromatic molecules, adding cheerfulness and bliss to the ambience of a romantic evening. A beautiful flower garden brightens the day with happiness and joy as it imparts its sweet, enchanting aromas for all to smell and delight in.

Enjoyable scents evoke our highest emotions. Our mind associates these scents with love, warmth, happiness, and comfort.

Since the beginning of time, people have been fond

of the exquisite fragrances of flowers and aromatic plants. These plant substances have been employed in various formulations for medicines and in foods. They have been used to scent the body, beautify the skin and hair, and uplift the spirit.

As early as 3000 B.C., the ancient Sumerians and Egyptians drenched themselves with a different scent on each part of their body daily. The hair was scented, and skin and nails were colored with a dye made from henna. Foods were scented and flavored, flower blossoms were strewn throughout households, statues were crowned with fragrant wreaths, and incense was burned in the streets during festivals.

Cleopatra, Queen of Egypt, had her feet rubbed with an ointment made from almonds, honey, cinnamon, and orange blossoms and her hands massaged with the oils of rose, saffron, and violet.

In order to seduce Mark Anthony, Cleopatra saturated the sails on her barge with floral fragrances and sat beneath a canopy that had garlands of roses while she waited to meet him. At the banquet, she had the floor carpeted with roses 18 inches (45 cm) high, held in nets. The air was heavy with incense, and each guest was crowned on arrival with a chaplet of flowers.

Wealthy ladies of ancient Greece and Rome had servants massage them with fragrant oils, and their hair washed and perfumed with these oils. A black powder, taken from burned incense, was used to darken their eyebrows and the edges of their eyelids.

In parts of Europe since medieval times, girls seeking a husband formulated a tonic of rose, violet, saffron, myrrh, lavender, and rosemary in the hope of improving their luck. Carnations were juiced and applied on the body as a perfume and the petals soaked in wine and drank as an aphrodisiac. Rosemary placed inside a pillow was believed to promote dreams of a future mate. Charms made with leaves of rosemary were thought to bring good luck for love and marriage.

Young European virgin girls were warned of their

vulnerability when smelling the fragrance of tuberose flowers in the presence of a male companion. This was thought to be especially true on a moonlit night, since the flowers emit a strong, sweet hypnotic scent after sundown. The Malayan people call the flower "mistress of the night."

A popular time and place for aromatics was sixteenth century England, during the reign of Queen Elizabeth I. Fragrant plants were used to scent linens; pillows and mattresses were stuffed with calming fragrances to provide a good night's sleep. Sachets containing dried leaves and flower petals were hung on chairs and bedposts. Lavender and mint flowers were scattered around homes to provide a fresh indoor scent and planted in gardens outside windows. Hair rinses were made with marigolds to add luster to the hair.

In nineteenth century Victorian England, wedding-flower bouquets were usually white to symbolize purity. White roses, orchids, carnations, orange blossoms, and the flowering branches of myrtle were favorites. A girl grew a myrtle bush and made a wreath to be worn on her wedding day.

In Europe and America, before the advent of synthetics and widely marketed commercial household goods, the stillroom was an important room for the woman of the house. In the quiet and peaceful atmosphere she dried, prepared, and stored the fragrant materials from the plants growing in the garden or from the wild. She made for the family: herbal medicines, cosmetics, aromatic candles and soaps, linen sachets, pillows, perfumes, potpourri, garlands, food flavorings and spices, and liqueurs. The recipes were passed from mother to daughter for generations and recorded in a recipe book.

In Asia and in the Pacific islands, women have been traditionally decorating and scenting the hair with fragrant flowers throughout the centuries. Women of Thailand adorn their hair with flowers for a sweet scent. Tagalog women of the Philippine

Islands condition their hair daily with coconut oil and an essence taken from flowers. Tahitian women mix coconut and sandalwood oils to beautify their skin and hair.

Jasmine flowers have been traditionally worn in the hair of Chinese women, who believed the enticing scent attracted men. Women from islands of the South Seas commonly wear hibiscus flowers. In Hawaii, vanda orchids are made into necklaces, or leis, and used as welcome and farewell gifts.

The flowers of rose, jasmine, violet, ylang-ylang, carnation and the spices of caraway, dill, clove, ginger, and galangal have all been major ingredients in love potions. Ylang-ylang flowers are recommended by doctors in India to help overcome frigidity and impotence. In Indonesia, ylang-ylang flowers are placed on the bed of newlyweds on their wedding night, and Hindu brides are anointed with jasmine oil.

In the mid-19th century, scientists began producing synthetic versions of essential oils, replacing these pure and precious natural substances that have been treasured for centuries.

Chemists are greatly skilled in their ability to create chemical compounds, reproducing scents that cost a fraction of the original, pure plant oils. These synthetic compounds, however, don't contain all the beneficial value of the plants. Also, the processing of these chemicals pollutes the earth, water, and air. Essential oils, on the other hand, are much more than just a fragrance. They are derived from plants, shrubs, trees, flowers, seeds, roots, and grasses and are the life force of the plants they are extracted from. These precious essences work on a much deeper level—affecting us not only in physical, but mental and spiritual, ways as well. They help balance our body, improve our well-being, and put us into greater harmony with the natural world.

When we blend these wonderful, pure, and natural oils, they can create enjoyable and effective products. The essences can be used for massage, skin and hair care, and as deodorants to keep fresh all day. Diffused or misted into the air, the blends can be made to smell like a sweet flower garden or the clean, fresh air of a lush evergreen forest. Relax to the satisfying pleasures of a calming bath, or, if you wish, become energized with a rejuvenating bath. There's also pet care, home care, personal care, and beauty care.

Make your own facial as well as skin and hair-care crèmes, hair rinses, after-bath moisturizers, body and foot powders, breath fresheners, bath oils, and bath salts. If you wish, you can make massage blends or fragrance your indoor environment by utilizing the aroma lamp, diffuser, lightbulb ring, and mist-spray formulas. In this book, there are over 540 formulas to select from, so surely you'll find ones that are just perfect for you. Treat yourself, your friends, and your loved ones to a more natural lifestyle, and enjoy the benefits of the essential oils to the fullest.

CHAPTER 1

Safe Use, Handling & Purity of Oils

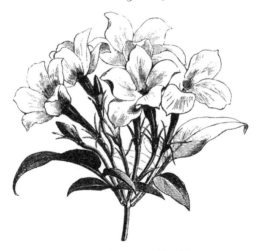

Jasmine (*Jasminum officinale*)

$\mathcal{E}$ssential oils are very concentrated substances and must be handled with care. Please follow these guidelines for safe and proper use.

- Before applying on the skin, dilute essential oils in a carrier oil, such as Almond (sweet), Grapeseed, Hazelnut, Jojoba, Kukui Nut, Macadamia Nut, or Sesame. This is necessary to prevent the possibility of any skin irritation. Should any irritation occur as a result of the essential oils, apply additional carrier oil. Lavender oil can also be used to quickly soothe the area.

 ❧ Take extra care not to get the oils or vapors in the eyes. If this occurs, flush with cool water.

 ❧ Many essential oils should not be used during pregnancy due to the stimulating effect they have on the urinary system and uterus. The oils can be helpful just before labor to facilitate the onset of childbirth. However, if used in the early months of pregnancy, they can bring on contractions, with the possibility of premature delivery.

Small amounts (2 to 3 drops at one time) of the following essential oils can be used during pregnancy: Bergamot, Coriander, Cypress, Frankincense, Geranium, Ginger, Grapefruit, Lavender, Lemon, Lime, Mandarin, Neroli, Orange, Patchouli, Petitgrain, Sandalwood, Spearmint, Tangerine, Tea Tree. Sesame oil can be used as a carrier oil.

§ If a woman is nursing her baby, she should use extra care in the selection of essential oils, especially for skin application, since the effects of the oils are transferred to the infant.

§ If a person is highly allergic, this simple and easy test can be done: First rub a drop of carrier oil on the upper chest area. In 12 hours check for redness on the skin or any other reaction. If the skin is clear, place 1 drop of an essential oil in 20 drops of the same carrier oil that was tested to be safe, and again rub the mixture on the upper chest. If there is no skin reaction after 12 hours, both the carrier and essential oil should be fine to use.

§ Do not consume alcohol, except for a small glass of wine with a meal, in the time period when using essential oils.

§ Do not use the essential oils while on medication since the oils might interfere with the medicine.

§ The following oils can be irritating to the skin. They must be used with extra care, particularly by people who have dry or sensitive skin: Anise, Basil (Sweet), Bay (West Indian), Bergamot, Birch (Sweet), Black Pepper, Cinnamon, Clove Bud, Fennel (Sweet), Ginger, Gingergrass, Grapefruit, Lemon, Lemongrass, Lime, Litsea Cubeba, Mandarin, Orange, Oregano, Peppermint, Pimento Berry, Pine, Spearmint, Tangerine, Thyme.

§ Avoid sitting in the sun, in tanning booths, or in the sauna or steam room for at least 4 hours after applying essential oils on the skin. Some essential oils are phototoxic.

Carefully read all precautions in chapter 8 (pp. 347–478).

❧ There are people with extremely sensitive skin who cannot tolerate the essential oils without having skin irritation. If this is the case, please discontinue use.

❧ The following essential oils should not be used by people prone to epileptic seizures: Fennel (Sweet), Hyssop Decumbens, Rosemary, Sage, Thyme.

❧ The following essential oils tend to slow down the reflexes and should be avoided before driving a vehicle or doing anything that requires full attention: Anise, Celery, Clary Sage, Dill, Elemi, Fennel (Sweet), Guaiacwood, Marjoram, Nutmeg.

❧ The following essential oils are stimulating and should be avoided before going to sleep: Cardamom, Eucalyptus, Ginger, Peppermint, Patchouli, Pine, Rosemary, Spearmint, Sage.

❧ When spilled on furniture, many essential oils will remove the finish; therefore, be careful when handling the bottles.

❧ Both light and oxygen cause oils to deteriorate rapidly. Refrigeration does not prevent spoilage, but it can diminish the speed at which it occurs. Kirlian photography has shown that violet-colored glass has an energizing effect on essential oil molecules and offers essential oils the best protection from light degradation, leading to increases to increased shelf life. Therefore, oils and blends should be stored in violet-colored glass bottles and jars and placed in a dark, cool area.

§ Use glass droppers when measuring drops of essential oil. See drop equivalents (p. 502).

§ Keep all bottles tightly closed to prevent the oils from evaporating and oxidizing.

§ After mixing carrier and essential oils together, use the blend as soon as possible, or within a six-month period, to avoid the possibility of spoilage.

§ Label all bottles and jars that contain blends.

§ Always store essential oils out of sight and the reach of children.

PURITY OF OILS

Before purchasing essential oils and carrier oils, it is important to become familiar with the different methods of extraction.

METHODS OF EXTRACTION FOR ESSENTIAL OILS

Steam Distillation: This method involves the use of steam from boiling water to release the volatile oils from the plant material. The steam is then cooled as it passes through a coil, which causes the steam to condense into a liquid. This liquid is composed of water and essential oil. The essential oil floats on top of the water and is skimmed off. The water is composed of water-soluble components from the oil and is used as floral water. This extraction method is most extensively used and produces a good-quality essential oil.

Carbon Dioxide Gas Extraction: There are two types of oil that are obtained from the carbon-dioxide (CO_2) extraction process. One is called *select;* the other is called *total.*

In the *select method,* the oil is extracted at a temperature of around 88° F (31° C). The plant material is placed in a chamber, and then the compressed CO_2 gas is released. As the gas passes through the plant material, it draws the plant components into solution. When the process is completed the pressure is lowered, and the extracted materials precipitate out and are collected. The CO_2 gas is then recompressed and recycled to be used again without leaving any residues in the extracted oil. The extracted oil contains selected components similar to the oils that are steam distilled.

In the *total extraction method,* the plant material is processed at a higher temperature. The extracted oil from this method contains more components than from the select method.

The CO_2 process equipment is extremely expensive, contributing to higher prices for the oils produced from this method.

Cold Pressed: Citrus oils are extracted from the peel of the fruit, using the cold-pressed method. The fruits are placed on a conveyor belt and then dropped into a cup with knives. As the cup closes, the knives puncture the fruit, releasing the water and oil. The liquid is then collected and put through a centrifuge that separates out the oil.

Maceration: This method involves the soaking of flowers, such as rose and jasmine, in hot oil to release the fragrant components into the oil.

METHODS OF EXTRACTION FOR CARRIER OILS

Expeller or Mechanically Pressed: Seeds, nuts, fruits, and vegetables are pressed without the use of heat. Temperatures can generally reach up to 185° F (85° C).

Cold Pressed: Oils are produced by a mechanical batch-pressing process in which heat-producing friction is minimized so that temperatures remain below 120° F (49° C). In-line refrigerated cooling devices are used on the expeller presses to keep the temperature down while the extraction is taking place.

These pressing methods are acceptable for producing good-quality oil. However, they are usually refined afterwards, using high heat and harsh chemicals. Therefore, it is important to check the label on the container to ensure that the oil is unrefined, containing all the valuable nutrients.

Solvent Extraction: Plant material is bathed in solvents, such as hexane and other toxic chemicals, to extract the oil. This method is less costly and yields a greater amount of oil. However, toxic residues remain in the oil. A high percentage of vegetable oils are solvent extracted. This is an unacceptable extraction method for people who seek pure oils.

SELECTING PURE OILS

The highest grade and most effective oils are produced from plants that grow in the wild, away from polluted sources, or from plants that are cultivated organically by natural farming methods. It is important to select for purchase unrefined cold-pressed, expeller-pressed, or mechanically pressed carrier oils and essential oils that have been steam distilled, CO_2 extracted, or cold pressed.

SHELF LIFE

The shelf life of most essential oils is about two to three years. Citrus oils, however, should be used within six to nine months. Blends have a shelf life of about six months. The shelf life for carrier oils is about one year. To extend the shelf life of carrier oils, store them in the freezer and refrigerate them after opening.

CHAPTER 2

Air Fragrances

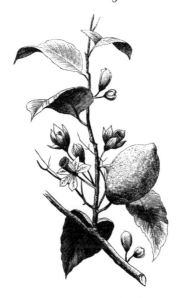

Lemon (*Citrus limon*)

$\mathcal{M}$any of us have experienced an elevated mood from smelling the beautiful scents of flowers and breathing the clean, fresh air in the forest. The essential oils allow us to recreate these wonderful atmospheres, providing us with scents we can enjoy and bring into our indoor environment to enhance our life.

Orange (*Citrus sinensis*)

AROMA LAMP

Select one of these formulas. Make sure the window(s) and door(s) in the room are closed to prevent the aromatic vapors from escaping. Fill the small container on top of the aroma lamp with purified water and add the essential oils. Depending on the type of aroma lamp you have, light the candle or turn on the lightbulb.

As the water heats, the aromatic vapors disperse into the air. Enjoy the fragrance!

ROOM FRAGRANCES

CITRUS SCENTS

Room Fragrance (Aroma Lamp)

Tangerine	20 drops
Lime	5 drops
Bergamot	5 drops
Cedarwood (Atlas)	5 drops

Room Fragrance (Aroma Lamp)

Orange	14 drops
Grapefruit	10 drops
Lemongrass	8 drops
Guaiacwood	3 drops

FLORAL SCENTS

Room Fragrance (Aroma Lamp)

Ylang-Ylang	20 drops
Lemon	7 drops
Clove Bud	5 drops
Lime	3 drops

Room Fragrance (Aroma Lamp)

Neroli	15 drops
Rose	10 drops
Ylang-Ylang	10 drops

Room Fragrance (Aroma Lamp)

Ylang-Ylang	15 drops
Neroli	10 drops
Petitgrain	5 drops
Orange	5 drops

Room Fragrance (Aroma Lamp)

Ylang-Ylang	22 drops
Geranium	5 drops
Lime	5 drops
Vanilla	3 drops

FOREST SCENTS

Room Fragrance (Aroma Lamp)

Spruce	20 drops
Rosemary	5 drops
Cedarwood (Atlas)	4 drops
Fennel (Sweet)	3 drops
Eucalyptus	3 drops

Room Fragrance (Aroma Lamp)

Cajeput	16 drops
Lavender	9 drops
Eucalyptus	5 drops
Fir Needles	5 drops

Mint Scents

Room Fragrance (Aroma Lamp)

| Peppermint | 32 drops |
| Cedarwood (Atlas) | 3 drops |

Room Fragrance (Aroma Lamp)

Spearmint	28 drops
Spruce	5 drops
Cedarwood (Atlas)	2 drops

Room Fragrance (Aroma Lamp)

Spearmint	22 drops
Clove Bud	6 drops
Lime	5 drops
Cedarwood (Atlas)	2 drops

SPICY SCENTS

Room Fragrance (Aroma Lamp)

Cinnamon Bark	20 drops
Orange	9 drops
Ginger	6 drops

Room Fragrance (Aroma Lamp)

Cinnamon Bark	20 drops
Tangerine	10 drops
Champaca Flower	5 drops

Room Fragrance (Aroma Lamp)

Cinnamon Bark	20 drops
Spearmint	9 drops
Spruce	6 drops

COTTON CLOTH

CLOTHES CLOSET FRESHENERS

In damp regions, moisture can cause clothes closets to taken on a disagreeable, stale, and musty smell. These formulas can help freshen the closet so that the clothes will smell nice.

Select one of these formulas. Place the drops of essential oils on a clean cotton cloth; then place the cloth in the closet. To avoid oil stains, make sure that it does not come into contact with any clothing. Place a scented cloth at each end of the closet. When the scent wears off, you can reapply the essential oils to the cloth.

Clothes Closet Freshener (Cotton Cloth)

Spearmint	50 drops
Amyris	20 drops

Clothes Closet Freshener (Cotton Cloth)

Orange	30 drops
Clove Bud	30 drops
Lavender	10 drops

Clothes Closet Freshener (Cotton Cloth)

Lemongrass	40 drops
Cedarwood (Atlas)	30 drops

Clothes Closet Freshener (Cotton Cloth)

Spearmint	40 drops
Orange	20 drops
Cassia Bark	10 drops

Clothes Closet Freshener (Cotton Cloth)

Litsea Cubeba	45 drops
Clove Bud	15 drops
Amyris	10 drops

Clothes Closet Freshener (Cotton Cloth)

Clove Bud	40 drops
Cedarwood (Atlas)	20 drops
Orange	10 drops

Clothes Closet Freshener (Cotton Cloth)

Peppermint	55 drops
Cabreuva	15 drops

CLOTHES DRAWER FRESHENERS

Place one of the formulas on a cotton cloth and fold it over several times. Wrap a second cloth around the first so that the oils do not come into contact with the clothes. Then place the cloth in the drawer and close it tightly so that the essential oil vapors do not escape. When the scent wears off, reapply the formula to the cloth.

Drawer Freshener (Cotton Cloth)

Spearmint	20 drops
Amyris	3 drops
Cabreuva	2 drops

Drawer Freshener (Cotton Cloth)

Spearmint	15 drops
Lavender	10 drops

Drawer Freshener (Cotton Cloth)
    Orange   12 drops
    Cassia Bark   10 drops
    Cedarwood (Atlas)   3 drops

Drawer Freshener (Cotton Cloth)
    Peppermint   20 drops
    Clove Bud   5 drops

Drawer Freshener (Cotton Cloth)
    Orange   20 drops
    Bergamot   5 drops

Drawer Freshener (Cotton Cloth)
    Lemongrass   13 drops
    Orange   10 drops
    Patchouli   2 drops

Drawer Freshener (Cotton Cloth)

Peppermint	15 drops
Basil (Sweet)	10 drops

Drawer Freshener (Cotton Cloth)

Bois de Rose	10 drops
Spearmint	10 drops
Cedarwood (Atlas)	5 drops

DIFFUSER

~

Diffusers disperse a mist of essential-oil microparticles, which create an aromatic atmosphere for the indoors. There are different types of diffusers on the market. You can choose a smaller or larger unit, depending on the size of the area to receive the fragrance.

The formulas in this section are given in percentages rather than drops because of the different types of units. One type requires essential oils to be placed on a pad. The unit warms the oils, dispersing the aroma into the air. Another type has a glass bottle into which essential oils are placed. The oil is then propelled into a nebulizer by air pressure and vaporized into the air. The third type of diffuser is fan driven. Cold water is poured into a slide-out container, and essential oils are added to the water. The fan disperses the aromatic vapors into the air.

Select one of these formulas. Make sure the window(s) and door(s) in the room are closed to prevent the aromatic vapors from escaping. Place the essential oils into the designated area of the diffuser, and turn on the unit to disperse the aroma. For large rooms, it is best to use a nebulizer diffuser.

LOCKER ROOM FRESHENERS

Locker Room Freshener (Diffuser)

Peppermint	50%
Bergamot	20%
Tangerine	20%
Cypress	10%

Locker Room Freshener (Diffuser)

Spearmint	50%
Grapefruit	30%
Lavender	10%
Niaouli	10%

Locker Room Freshener (Diffuser)

Lemongrass	50%
Tangerine	40%
Bay (West Indian)	10%

Locker Room Freshener (Diffuser)

Peppermint	70%
Bay (West Indian)	20%
Cinnamon Leaf	10%

Locker Room Freshener (Diffuser)

Spearmint	40%
Eucalyptus	20%
Cabreuva	20%
Cajeput	20%

Locker Room Freshener (Diffuser)

Tangerine	40%
Grapefruit	40%
Cinnamon Bark	20%

REMOVE FOUL ODORS

Remove Foul Odors (Diffuser)

Peppermint	30%
Bois de Rose	30%
Lemongrass	20%
Clove Bud	20%

Remove Foul Odors (Diffuser)

Litsea Cubeba	30%
Orange	30%
Cinnamon Bark	20%
Grapefruit	20%

ROOM DISINFECTANTS

Room Disinfectant (Diffuser)

Ravensara Aromatica	50%
Lavender	30%
Lemongrass	20%

Room Disinfectant (Diffuser)

Bergamot	30%
Cajeput	30%
Clove Bud	20%
Cinnamon Leaf	20%

Room Disinfectant (Diffuser)

Lemon	80%
Peppermint	20%

Room Disinfectant (Diffuser)

Cinnamon Bark	40%
Orange	40%
Ginger	20%

ROOM FRAGRANCES

CITRUS SCENTS

Room Fragrance (Diffuser)

Tangerine	50%
Lemongrass	40%
Bergamot	10%

Room Fragrance (Diffuser)

Orange	30%
Grapefruit	30%
Lemon	30%
Petitgrain	10%

FLORAL SCENTS

Room Fragrance (Diffuser)

Ylang-Ylang	50%
Geranium	20%
Lemon	10%
Petitgrain	10%
Clove Bud	10%

Room Fragrance (Diffuser)

Neroli	40%
Ylang-Ylang	40%
Bergamot	10%
Bay (West Indian)	10%

Forest Scents

Room Fragrance (Diffuser)

Spruce	40%
Juniper Berry	30%
Fir Needles	20%
Peppermint	10%

Room Fragrance (Diffuser)

Spruce	70%
Cajeput	10%
Pine	10%
Eucalyptus	10%

MINT SCENTS

Room Fragrance (Diffuser)

Peppermint	80%
Lavender	20%

Room Fragrance (Diffuser)

Spearmint	90%
Spruce	10%

Room Fragrance (Diffuser)

Spearmint	70%
Lime	20%
Clove Bud	10%

SPICY SCENTS

Room Fragrance (Diffuser)

Cinnamon Bark	50%
Orange	30%
Ginger	20%

Room Fragrance (Diffuser)

Lemon	60%
Clove Bud	30%
Sage (Spanish)	10%

Room Fragrance (Diffuser)

Tangerine	40%
Thyme	30%
Lemon	30%

FRAGRANCE JAR

Select one of these formulas. Make sure the window(s) and door(s) in the room are closed to prevent the aromatic vapors from escaping. Combine the essential oils in the fragrance jar; then put the cork in the opening of the jar. Gently shake the jar to mix the oils well. Place the jar nearby in order to enjoy the aroma as it diffuses from around the cork and through the clay terra-cotta material. Loosen the cork if you desire a stronger aroma to be diffused.

Room Fragrances

Citrus Scents

Room Fragrance (Fragrance Jar)

Litsea Cubeba	30 drops
Grapefruit	10 drops
Lemon	10 drops

Room Fragrance (Fragrance Jar)

Lime	20 drops
Lemon	15 drops
Bergamot	15 drops

FLORAL SCENTS

Room Fragrance (Fragrance Jar)

Champaca Flower	20 drops
Rose	10 drops
Bergamot	10 drops
Geranium	10 drops

Room Fragrance (Fragrance Jar)

Champaca Flower	20 drops
Ylang-Ylang	20 drops
Vanilla	10 drops

FOREST SCENTS

Room Fragrance (Fragrance Jar)

Spruce	30 drops
Eucalyptus	10 drops
Lavender	10 drops

Room Fragrance (Fragrance Jar)

Cajeput	15 drops
Spruce	15 drops
Fir Needles	10 drops
Ravensara Aromatica	5 drops
Amyris	5 drops

MINT SCENTS

Room Fragrance (Fragrance Jar)

Peppermint	25 drops
Ravensara Aromatica	10 drops
Juniper Berry	10 drops
Lavender	5 drops

Room Fragrance (Fragrance Jar)

Spearmint	25 drops
Lime	10 drops
Bergamot	10 drops
Pimento Berry	5 drops

~

SPICY SCENTS

Room Fragrance (Fragrance Jar)

Cinnamon Bark	25 drops
Clove Bud	15 drops
Peppermint	10 drops

Room Fragrance (Fragrance Jar)

Pimento Berry	25 drops
Lime	15 drops
Clove Bud	10 drops

Room Fragrance (Fragrance Jar)

Cinnamon Bark	25 drops
Spruce	25 drops

Room Fragrance (Fragrance Jar)

Basil (Sweet)	20 drops
Bergamot	20 drops
Thyme	10 drops

LIGHTBULB RING

Select one of these formulas. Make sure the window(s) and door(s) in the room are closed to prevent the aromatic vapors from escaping. Place the lightbulb ring on top of a cool lightbulb and carefully drop the essential oils into the circular groove of the ring. Avoid getting any oil on the lightbulb. Turn on the light and, as the bulb heats the oils, the aromatic fragrance will be diffused into the air. Use only lightbulbs of 60 watts or less.

ROOM FRAGRANCES

CITRUS SCENTS

Room Fragrance (Lightbulb Ring)

Lemongrass	6 drops
Lime	4 drops
Tangerine	3 drops
Patchouli	2 drops

Room Fragrance (Lightbulb Ring)

Litsea Cubeba	10 drops
Grapefruit	4 drops
Cinnamon Leaf	1 drop

FLORAL SCENTS

Room Fragrance (Lightbulb Ring)

Rose	11 drops
Orange	4 drops

Room Fragrance (Lightbulb Ring)

Neroli	6 drops
Bergamot	4 drops
Champaca Flower	3 drops
Petitgrain	2 drops

Room Fragrance (Lightbulb Ring)

Litsea Cubeba	5 drops
Ylang-Ylang	4 drops
Lavender	4 drops
Helichrysum	1 drop
Geranium	1 drop

Forest Scents

Room Fragrance (Lightbulb Ring)

Spruce	10 drops
Cedarwood (Atlas)	3 drops
Juniper Berry	2 drops

Room Fragrance (Lightbulb Ring)

Fir Needles	10 drops
Pine	2 drops
Spruce	2 drops
Cedarwood (Atlas)	1 drop

MINT SCENTS

Room Fragrance (Lightbulb Ring)

Spearmint	11 drops
Peppermint	3 drops
Patchouli	1 drop

Room Fragrance (Lightbulb Ring)

Peppermint	13 drops
Copaiba	2 drops

Room Fragrance (Lightbulb Ring)

Spearmint	10 drops
Lime	5 drops

Spicy Scents

Room Fragrance (Lightbulb Ring)

Cinnamon Bark	10 drops
Vanilla	5 drops

Room Fragrance (Lightbulb Ring)

Cinnamon Bark	10 drops
Champaca Flower	3 drops
Geranium	1 drop
Patchouli	1 drop

Room Fragrance (Lightbulb Ring)

Cinnamon Bark	10 drops
Spruce	3 drops
Lavender	2 drops

Room Fragrance (Lightbulb Ring)

Cinnamon Leaf	13 drops
Peppermint	2 drops

MIST SPRAYS

Select one of these formulas. Make sure the window(s) and door(s) in the room are closed to prevent the aromatic vapors from escaping.

Fill a fine-mist-spray glass bottle with 4 fluid ounces (120 ml) of purified water, add the essential oils, tighten the cap, and shake well. Set aside for a day. As the aromas mature in the bottle, the fragrance improves and becomes stronger.

To use: Shake well again, and spray the mist into the air numerous times. Store in a dark, cool place.

LOCKER ROOM FRESHENERS

Locker Room Freshener (Mist Spray)

Peppermint	80 drops
Cajeput	40 drops
Litsea Cubeba	30 drops
Patchouli	10 drops
Pure Water	4 fl oz (120 ml)

Locker Room Freshener (Mist Spray)

Spearmint	75 drops
Spruce	40 drops
Cedarwood (Atlas)	30 drops
Lemon	15 drops
Pure Water	4 fl oz (120 ml)

Locker Room Freshener (Mist Spray)

Lemongrass	70 drops
Tangerine	60 drops
Bay (West Indian)	20 drops
Copaiba	10 drops
Pure Water	4 fl oz (120 ml)

Locker Room Freshener (Mist Spray)

Peppermint	70 drops
Bay (West Indian)	30 drops
Cinnamon Leaf	30 drops
Cedarwood (Atlas)	30 drops
Pure Water	4 fl oz (120 ml)

Locker Room Freshener (Mist Spray)

Clove Bud	50 drops
Lemongrass	50 drops
Orange	30 drops
Grapefruit	30 drops
Pure Water	4 fl oz (120 ml)

REMOVE FOUL ODORS

These mist-spray formulas can be very helpful to freshen any area of the house, especially odors from soiled diapers, the garbage, and the bathroom.

Remove Foul Odors (Mist Spray)

Lemongrass	85 drops
Spruce	40 drops
Pine	20 drops
Cedarwood (Atlas)	20 drops
Patchouli	10 drops
Pure Water	4 fl oz (120 ml)

Remove Foul Odors (Mist Spray)

Lavender	50 drops
Spearmint	50 drops
Amyris	40 drops
Spruce	35 drops
Pure Water	4 fl oz (120 ml)

Remove Foul Odors (Mist Spray)

Lemon	40 drops
Cinnamon Leaf	40 drops
Copaiba	40 drops
Peppermint	35 drops
Lemongrass	20 drops
Pure Water	4 fl oz (120 ml)

Remove Foul Odors (Mist Spray)

Grapefruit	60 drops
Litsea Cubeba	60 drops
Clove Bud	30 drops
Copaiba	15 drops
Patchouli	10 drops
Pure Water	4 fl oz (120 ml)

Room Disinfectants

Room Disinfectant (Mist Spray)

Bergamot	60 drops
Oregano	40 drops
Lavender	25 drops
Spearmint	25 drops
Cedarwood (Atlas)	15 drops
Cinnamon Leaf	10 drops
Pure Water	4 fl oz (120 ml)

Room Disinfectant (Mist Spray)

Cajeput	40 drops
Bergamot	40 drops
Peppermint	40 drops
Clove Bud	20 drops
Tea Tree	20 drops
Copaiba	15 drops
Pure Water	4 fl oz (120 ml)

Room Disinfectant (Mist Spray)

Thyme	40 drops
Cinnamon Leaf	40 drops
Lavender	40 drops
Lemon	40 drops
Copaiba	15 drops
Pure Water	4 fl oz (120 ml)

Room Disinfectant (Mist Spray)

Oregano	50 drops
Lavender	50 drops
Pimento Berry	40 drops
Lime	35 drops
Pure Water	4 fl oz (120 ml)

ROOM FRAGRANCES

CITRUS SCENTS

Room Fragrance (Mist Spray)

Lime	90 drops
Tangerine	50 drops
Grapefruit	30 drops
Guaiacwood	5 drops
Pure Water	4 fl oz (120 ml)

Room Fragrance (Mist Spray)

Grapefruit	75 drops
Orange	60 drops
Litsea Cubeba	30 drops
Cedarwood (Atlas)	10 drops
Pure Water	4 fl oz (120 ml)

Room Fragrance (Mist Spray)

Lime	60 drops
Bergamot	60 drops
Tangerine	30 drops
Petitgrain	15 drops
Patchouli	10 drops
Pure Water	4 fl oz (120 ml)

Room Fragrance (Mist Spray)

Lemongrass	80 drops
Lemon	60 drops
Ginger	20 drops
Orange	15 drops
Pure Water	4 fl oz (120 ml)

FLORAL SCENTS

Room Fragrance (Mist Spray)

Ylang-Ylang	80 drops
Petitgrain	30 drops
Neroli	25 drops
Clove Bud	15 drops
Pure Water	4 fl oz (120 ml)

Room Fragrance (Mist Spray)

Neroli	50 drops
Rose	50 drops
Orange	25 drops
Vanilla	25 drops
Pure Water	4 fl oz (120 ml)

Room Fragrance (Mist Spray)

Ylang-Ylang	80 drops
Champaca Flower	40 drops
Grapefruit	30 drops
Pure Water	4 fl oz (120 ml)

Room Fragrance (Mist Spray)

Neroli	50 drops
Ylang-Ylang	50 drops
Bergamot	35 drops
Petitgrain	15 drops
Pure Water	4 fl oz (120 ml)

Forest Scents

Room Fragrance (Mist Spray)

Spruce	60 drops
Juniper Berry	55 drops
Sandalwood	35 drops
Pure Water	4 fl oz (120 ml)

Room Fragrance (Mist Spray)

Cajeput	60 drops
Cinnamon Leaf	35 drops
Spruce	30 drops
Vanilla	10 drops
Amyris	10 drops
Fennel (Sweet)	5 drops
Pure Water	4 fl oz (120 ml)

Room Fragrance (Mist Spray)

Spruce	65 drops
Eucalyptus	35 drops
Bay (West Indian)	20 drops
Lime	10 drops
Lavender	10 drops
Cedarwood (Atlas)	10 drops
Pure Water	4 fl oz (120 ml)

Room Fragrance (Mist Spray)

Cajeput	50 drops
Fir Needles	35 drops
Spruce	30 drops
Sandalwood	20 drops
Spearmint	15 drops
Pure Water	4 fl oz (120 ml)

Mint Scents

Room Fragrance (Mist Spray)

Peppermint	90 drops
Spearmint	30 drops
Cinnamon Leaf	25 drops
Patchouli	5 drops
Pure Water	4 fl oz (120 ml)

Room Fragrance (Mist Spray)

Spearmint	80 drops
Peppermint	40 drops
Lavender	20 drops
Copaiba	10 drops
Pure Water	4 fl oz (120 ml)

Room Fragrance (Mist Spray)

Peppermint	80 drops
Cinnamon Leaf	30 drops
Vanilla	20 drops
Lavender	20 drops
Pure Water	4 fl oz (120 ml)

Room Fragrance (Mist Spray)

Spearmint	85 drops
Eucalyptus	30 drops
Peppermint	25 drops
Sandalwood	10 drops
Pure Water	4 fl oz (120 ml)

SPICY SCENTS

Room Fragrance (Mist Spray)

Orange	40 drops
Bay (West Indian)	40 drops
Clove Bud	30 drops
Cinnamon Leaf	30 drops
Vanilla	10 drops
Pure Water	4 fl oz (120 ml)

Room Fragrance (Mist Spray)

Cinnamon Leaf	40 drops
Pimento Berry	35 drops
Clove Bud	20 drops
Spruce	20 drops
Copaiba	20 drops
Spearmint	15 drops
Pure Water	4 fl oz (120 ml)

POTPOURRI POT

Select one of these formulas. Make sure the window(s) and door(s) in the room are closed to prevent the aromatic vapors from escaping.

Fill the empty potpourri pot about one-third full with purified water, add the essential oils, and heat to diffuse the aroma into the air. When you are finished diffusing the oils in the pot, pour the remaining aromatic water into a fine-mist-spray bottle; add fresh oils, and use as a mist spray.

ROOM FRAGRANCES

CITRUS SCENTS

Room Fragrance (Potpourri Pot)

Lime	20 drops
Lemon	10 drops
Grapefruit	10 drops
Cedarwood (Atlas)	5 drops

Room Fragrance (Potpourri Pot)

Tangerine	20 drops
Orange	10 drops
Lemongrass	10 drops
Champaca Flower	5 drops

FLORAL SCENTS

Room Fragrance (Potpourri Pot)

Vanilla	15 drops
Champaca Flower	10 drops
Bergamot	10 drops
Neroli	10 drops

Room Fragrance (Potpourri Pot)

Vanilla	10 drops
Ylang-Ylang	10 drops
Neroli	10 drops
Rose	10 drops
Geranium	5 drops

FOREST SCENTS

Room Fragrance (Potpourri Pot)

Spruce	25 drops
Juniper Berry	8 drops
Lavender	7 drops
Copaiba	5 drops

Room Fragrance (Potpourri Pot)

Ravensara Aromatica	15 drops
Spruce	15 drops
Fir Needles	10 drops
Copaiba	5 drops

MINT SCENTS

Room Fragrance (Potpourri Pot)

Peppermint	40 drops
Copaiba	5 drops

Room Fragrance (Potpourri Pot)

Spearmint	35 drops
Cabreuva	5 drops
Eucalyptus	5 drops

Spicy Scents

Room Fragrance (Potpourri Pot)

Cinnamon Bark	20 drops
Pimento Berry	10 drops
Bergamot	10 drops
Vanilla	5 drops

Room Fragrance (Potpourri Pot)

Cinnamon Bark	22 drops
Clove Bud	12 drops
Spruce	8 drops
Copaiba	3 drops

CHAPTER 3

Bath, Beauty & Personal Care

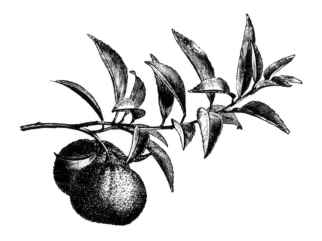

Mandarin Orange (*Citrus nobilis*)

To many people, it is becoming more apparent everyday that pure and natural products are best for us and for our loved ones to use. Now you can purchase quality ingredients and make your own natural products in a short period of time. Most of the formulas only take a few minutes to blend. Knowing that you made these products yourself, you and your family will enjoy using them so much more.

BATH OILS

❧

Soaking in warm water scented with essential oils can be so pleasurable that once you experience an aromatic bath, plain water baths will become a thing of the past.

Select one of these formulas. Combine the oils in a small glass bottle. Close the bathroom window and door. Fill the bathtub with water, as warm as you like, and pour the bath-oil formula into the bathwater. Swirl the water to distribute the oils evenly throughout the tub. Enter the bath immediately to capture all the benefits of the essential oils. Relax for thirty minutes.

CALMING

Calming Bath Oil

Ylang-Ylang	4 drops
Champaca Flower	4 drops
Neroli	4 drops
Petitgrain	3 drops
Carrier Oil	1 t (5 ml)

Calming Bath Oil

Manuka	5 drops
Spruce	5 drops
Marjoram	3 drops
Anise	2 drops
Carrier Oil	1 t (5 ml)

Calming Bath Oil

Vanilla	6 drops
Sandalwood	5 drops
Geranium	4 drops
Carrier Oil	1 t (5 ml)

Calming Bath Oil

Vanilla	5 drops
Mandarin	4 drops
Vetiver	3 drops
Petitgrain	3 drops
Carrier Oil	1 t (5 ml)

Calming Bath Oil

Frankincense	5 drops
Spruce	5 drops
St.-John's-Wort	5 drops
Carrier Oil	1 t (5 ml)

Calming Bath Oil

St.-John's-Wort	5 drops
Chamomile	4 drops
Guaiacwood	3 drops
Neroli	3 drops
Carrier Oil	1 t (5 ml)

PMS EASE

PMS-Ease Bath Oil

Caraway	5 drops
Vanilla	4 drops
Petitgrain	4 drops
Fennel (Sweet)	2 drops
Carrier Oil	1 t (5 ml)

PMS-Ease Bath Oil

Cypress	4 drops
Fennel (Sweet)	4 drops
Lavender	4 drops
Petitgrain	3 drops
Carrier Oil	1 t (5 ml)

PMS-Ease Bath Oil

Neroli	4 drops
Mandarin	4 drops
Lavender	4 drops
Rose	3 drops
Carrier Oil	1 t (5 ml)

PMS-Ease Bath Oil

Helichrysum	4 drops
Dill	4 drops
Mandarin	4 drops
Petitgrain	3 drops
Carrier Oil	1 t (5 ml)

PMS-Ease Bath Oil

Vanilla	5 drops
Neroli	4 drops
Petitgrain	4 drops
Dill	2 drops
Carrier Oil	1 t (5 ml)

PMS-Ease Bath Oil

Vanilla	5 drops
Mandarin	4 drops
Juniper Berry	3 drops
Frankincense	3 drops
Carrier Oil	1 t (5 ml)

REJUVENATING

Rejuvenating Bath Oil

Fir Needles	5 drops
Eucalyptus	5 drops
Spearmint	3 drops
Cabreuva	2 drops
Carrier Oil	1 t (5 ml)

Rejuvenating Bath Oil

Rosemary	5 drops
Hyssop Decumbens	4 drops
Peppermint	3 drops
Helichrysum	3 drops
Carrier Oil	1 t (5 ml)

Rejuvenating Bath Oil

Cabreuva	5 drops
Eucalyptus	5 drops
Grapefruit	3 drops
Spearmint	2 drops
Carrier Oil	1 t (5 ml)

Rejuvenating Bath Oil

Helichrysum	6 drops
Spruce	4 drops
Cabreuva	3 drops
Lemon	2 drops
Carrier Oil	1 t (5 ml)

BATH SALTS

Select one of these formulas. Measure and pour the sea salt into a widemouthed glass jar, add the essential oils, and mix well. Then place the cap on the jar and tighten. Close the bathroom window and door. Fill the bathtub with water, as warm as you like, and pour the bath-salt formula into the bathwater. Swirl the water to dissolve and distribute the salt and to prevent it from settling on the bottom of the tub.

Be careful when you get into the tub, since undissolved salt crystals can make the tub surface slippery. Enter the bath immediately to capture all the benefits of the essential oils. Relax for thirty minutes.

Helpful Measurement: 1 cup (240 ml) of sea salt weighs about 10 ounces or 284 grams.

BREATHE MORE EASILY

People who live in large cities generally take shallow breaths, since the air is so polluted. Breathing deeply is a healthy practice. Use these bath salts to help encourage deep breathing.

Breathe More Easily Bath Salts

Sea Salt	1 cup (284 g)
Manuka	5 drops
Litsea Cubeba	4 drops
Lavender	4 drops
Niaouli	2 drops

Breathe More Easily Bath Salts

Sea Salt	1 cup (284 g)
Cajeput	4 drops
Lavender	4 drops
Copaiba	4 drops
Spearmint	3 drops

Breathe More Easily Bath Salts

Sea Salt	1 cup (284 g)
Lavender	5 drops
Sandalwood	5 drops
Ravensara Aromatica	3 drops
Geranium	2 drops

Breathe More Easily Bath Salts

Sea Salt	1 cup (284 g)
Sandalwood	6 drops
Copaiba	3 drops
Litsea Cubeba	3 drops
Spruce	3 drops

CALMING

Helpful Measurement: 1 cup (240 ml) of Epsom salts weighs about 10 ounces or 284 grams.

Calming Bath Salts

Epsom Salts	1 cup (284 g)
Neroli	6 drops
Petitgrain	5 drops
Ylang-Ylang	4 drops

Calming Bath Salts

Epsom Salts	1 cup (284 g)
Amyris	7 drops
Clary Sage	3 drops
Anise	3 drops
Tangerine	2 drops

Rejuvenating

Rejuvenating Bath Salts

Sea Salt	1 cup (284 g)
Fir Needles	4 drops
Rosemary	4 drops
Spearmint	3 drops
Sage (Spanish)	2 drops
Litsea Cubeba	2 drops

Rejuvenating Bath Salts

Sea Salt	1 cup (284 g)
Spruce	6 drops
Helichrysum	6 drops
Peppermint	3 drops

Rejuvenating Bath Salts

Sea Salt	1 cup (284 g)
Ravensara Aromatica	5 drops
Eucalyptus	3 drops
Spearmint	3 drops
Lime	2 drops
Hyssop Decumbens	2 drops

FOOTBATHS

Select one of these formulas. Fill a basin with warm water. Mix the essential oils into a carrier oil, such as sweet almond, hazelnut, or sesame, and add the formula to the water. Swirl the water to disperse the oils throughout and soak the feet for thirty minutes.

REJUVENATING

Rejuvenating Footbath

Grapefruit	6 drops
Lemon	5 drops
Ginger	4 drops
Carrier Oil	1 t (5 ml)

Rejuvenating Footbath

Rosemary	4 drops
Lemon	4 drops
Helichrysum	4 drops
Cabreuva	3 drops
Carrier Oil	1 t (5 ml)

Rejuvenating Footbath

Eucalyptus	5 drops
Spearmint	4 drops
Niaouli	4 drops
Hyssop Decumbens	2 drops
Carrier Oil	1 t (5 ml)

Rejuvenating Footbath

Grapefruit	6 drops
Cabreuva	5 drops
Spearmint	2 drops
Sage (Spanish)	2 drops
Carrier Oil	1 t (5 ml)

Rejuvenating Footbath

Cabreuva	5 drops
Spearmint	4 drops
Coriander	3 drops
Niaouli	3 drops
Carrier Oil	1 t (5 ml)

Rejuvenating Footbath

Peppermint	5 drops
Fir Needles	5 drops
Sage (Spanish)	3 drops
Copaiba	2 drops
Carrier Oil	1 t (5 ml)

RELAXING

Relaxing Footbath

Spruce	7 drops
Frankincense	5 drops
Cinnamon Leaf	3 drops
Carrier Oil	1 t (5 ml)

Relaxing Footbath

Orange	5 drops
Juniper Berry	4 drops
Lavender	3 drops
Bergamot	3 drops
Carrier Oil	1 t (5 ml)

Relaxing Footbath

Petitgrain	6 drops
Neroli	6 drops
Guaiacwood	3 drops
Carrier Oil	1 t (5 ml)

Relaxing Footbath

Spruce	5 drops
Vanilla	4 drops
Lemongrass	4 drops
Cedarwood (Atlas)	2 drops
Carrier Oil	1 t (5 ml)

Relaxing Footbath

Orange	5 drops
Cajeput	5 drops
Vetiver	3 drops
Chamomile	2 drops
Carrier Oil	1 t (5 ml)

Relaxing Footbath

Neroli	6 drops
Ylang-Ylang	5 drops
Sandalwood	4 drops
Carrier Oil	1 t (5 ml)

SAUNA & STEAM ROOM
Breathe More Easily

Select one of these formulas. Fill a fine-mist-spray glass bottle with 4 fluid ounces (120 ml) of purified water. Add the essential oils, tighten the cap, and shake well.

To use: Shake well. While entering the sauna or steam room, spray the mist several times away from the face and body to avoid getting any essential oil droplets on the skin. Then relax for about 10 minutes at a time and enjoy the aroma.

Repeat use of the mist when needed or desired.

Sauna & Steam Room (Mist Spray)

Fir Needles	60 drops
Spruce	60 drops
Spearmint	20 drops
Juniper Berry	10 drops
Pure Water	4 fl oz (120 ml)

Sauna & Steam Room (Mist Spray)

Eucalyptus	60 drops
Lavender	60 drops
Vanilla	20 drops
Juniper Berry	10 drops
Pure Water	4 fl oz (120 ml)

Sauna & Steam Room (Mist Spray)

Spruce	60 drops
Lavender	40 drops
Cajeput	30 drops
Pine	20 drops
Pure Water	4 fl oz (120 ml)

Sauna & Steam Room (Mist Spray)

Lavender	65 drops
Fir Needles	50 drops
Niaouli	30 drops
Cedarwood (Atlas)	5 drops
Pure Water	4 fl oz (120 ml)

FACIAL CRÈMES

Select one of these formulas. Place the shea butter into a widemouthed glass jar and put the jar in a small cooking pot of water. Heat on a low flame. When the butter has melted, add the jojoba oil and stir well. Remove the jar from the heated water, and, as the ingredients cool, mix the essential oils in well. Then place the cap on the jar and tighten. Let the crème sit for several hours until it becomes creamy in texture.

Use an ample amount to moisturize your skin. Store in a dark, cool place.

Helpful Measurement: 2 tablespoons (30 ml) of shea butter weighs about 1 ounce or 28 grams.

Facial Crème

Sandalwood	20 drops
Rose	10 drops
Shea Butter	2 T (28 g)
Jojoba	8 t (40 ml)

Facial Crème

Rose	12 drops
Bois de Rose	10 drops
Copaiba	8 drops
Shea Butter	2 T (28 g)
Jojoba	8 t (40 ml)

Facial Crème

Sandalwood	13 drops
Neroli	12 drops
Petitgrain	5 drops
Shea Butter	2 T (28 g)
Jojoba	8 t (40 ml)

Facial Crème

Tangerine	16 drops
Vetiver	10 drops
Palmarosa	4 drops
Shea Butter	2 T (28 g)
Jojoba	8 t (40 ml)

HAIR & SCALP MOISTURIZING CRÈMES

Select one of these formulas. Place the shea butter into a widemouthed glass jar and put the jar in a small cooking pot of water. Heat on a low flame. When the butter has melted, add the jojoba oil and stir well. Remove the jar from the heated water, and, as the ingredients cool, mix the essential oils in well. Then place the cap on the jar and tighten. Let the crème sit for several hours until it becomes creamy in texture.

To use: Dampen the hair with water, apply the necessary amount of crème, rub well into the scalp, then brush or comb the crème through the hair. Store in a dark, cool place.

Helpful Measurement: 2 tablespoons (30 ml) of shea butter weighs about 1 ounce or 28 grams.

Hair & Scalp Moisturizing Crème

Sandalwood	25 drops
Peppermint	15 drops
Shea Butter	2 T (28 g)
Jojoba	3 T (45 ml)

Hair & Scalp Moisturizing Crème

Sandalwood	25 drops
Ylang-Ylang	15 drops
Shea Butter	2 T (28 g)
Jojoba	3 T (45 ml)

Hair & Scalp Moisturizing Crème

Copaiba	20 drops
Vanilla	15 drops
Bois de Rose	5 drops
Shea Butter	2 T (28 g)
Jojoba	3 T (45 ml)

Hair & Scalp Moisturizing Crème

Rose	20 drops
Sandalwood	10 drops
Petitgrain	10 drops
Shea Butter	2 T (28 g)
Jojoba	3 T (45 ml)

Hair Rinses

Select one of these formulas. Mix the ingredients in a glass bottle. Shake well and apply a small portion on the scalp and hair after washing the hair. Avoid getting the hair rinse near or in the eyes. Towel dry. If you wish to scent the hair afterward, use one of the body-mist formulas (pp. 145–147).

To store: Place a label on the hair-rinse bottle and refrigerate. For the next use, warm the portion of the rinse that will be used.

Hair Rinse

Peppermint	10 drops
Copaiba	10 drops
Lavender	5 drops
Aloe Vera Juice	2 T (30 ml)
Apple Cider Vinegar	1 T (15 ml)
Pure Water	3½ cups (0.84 L)

Hair Rinse

Sandalwood	18 drops
Ylang-Ylang	7 drops
Aloe Vera Juice	2 T (30 ml)
Apple Cider Vinegar	1 T (15 ml)
Pure Water	3½ cups (0.84 L)

Hair Rinse

Helichrysum	13 drops
Spearmint	10 drops
Lavender	2 drops
Aloe Vera Juice	2 T (30 ml)
Apple Cider Vinegar	1 T (15 ml)
Pure Water	3½ cups (0.84 L)

Hair Rinse

Niaouli	10 drops
Vanilla	10 drops
Lavender	5 drops
Aloe Vera Juice	2 T (30 ml)
Apple Cider Vinegar	1 T (15 ml)
Pure Water	3½ cups (0.84 L)

SKIN-CARE CRÈMES

Select one of these formulas. Place the shea butter into a widemouthed glass jar and put the jar in a small cooking pot of water. Heat on a low flame. When the butter melts, add the jojoba oil and stir well. Remove the jar from the heated water, and as the ingredients cool, mix the essential oils in well. Then place the cap on the jar and tighten. Let the crème sit for several hours until it becomes creamy in texture.

Apply an ample amount to moisturize your skin. Store in a dark, cool place.

Helpful Measurement: 2 tablespoons (30 ml) of shea butter weighs about 1 ounce or 28 grams.

Skin-Care Crème

Sandalwood	35 drops
Elemi	15 drops
Shea Butter	2 T (28 g)
Jojoba	8 t (40 ml)

Skin-Care Crème

Sandalwood	30 drops
Rose	15 drops
Mandarin	5 drops
Shea Butter	2 T (28 g)
Jojoba	8 t (40 ml)

Skin-Care Crème

Helichrysum	30 drops
Amyris	10 drops
Ylang-Ylang	10 drops
Shea Butter	2 T (28 g)
Jojoba	8 t (40 ml)

Skin-Care Crème

Labdanum (Cistus)	15 drops
Vanilla	15 drops
Petitgrain	10 drops
Rose	10 drops
Shea Butter	2 T (28 g)
Jojoba	8 t (40 ml)

AFTER-BATH SKIN MOISTURIZERS

Select one of these formulas. Place the cocoa butter into a widemouthed glass jar, and put the jar in a small cooking pot of water. Heat on a low flame. When the cocoa butter melts, add the jojoba oil and stir well. Remove the jar from the heated water, and, as the ingredients cool, mix the essential oils in well. Then place the cap on the jar and tighten. Let the crème sit for several hours until it becomes creamy in texture.

Use as a skin moisturizer after your bath. Store in a dark, cool place.

Helpful Measurements: 7 teaspoons (35 ml) of cocoa butter weighs about 24.5 grams, a little less than 1 ounce.

After-Bath Skin Moisturizer

Sandalwood	20 drops
Neroli	5 drops
Rose	5 drops
Cocoa Butter	7 t (24.5 g)
Jojoba	2 t (10 ml)

After-Bath Skin Moisturizer

Elemi	15 drops
Vanilla	10 drops
Frankincense	5 drops
Cocoa Butter	7 t (24.5 g)
Jojoba	2 t (10 ml)

After-Bath Skin Moisturizer

Vanilla	15 drops
Sandalwood	15 drops
Cocoa Butter	7 t (24.5 g)
Jojoba	2 t (10 ml)

After-Bath Skin Moisturizer

Sandalwood	15 drops
Elemi	10 drops
Copaiba	5 drops
Cocoa Butter	7 t (24.5 g)
Jojoba	2 t (10 ml)

BODY SCENTING

BODY MISTS

Select one of these body-scenting formulas. Fill a fine-mist-spray glass bottle with 2 fluid ounces (60 ml) of purified water, add the essential oils, tighten the cap, and shake well. Before using, shake again and mist the body to impart fragrance to the skin and hair. Avoid getting the vapors near or in the eyes.

As the oils age in the bottle, the fragrance will improve. Store in a dark, cool place.

Body-Scenting Mist

Ylang-Ylang	10 drops
Vanilla	10 drops
Sandalwood	10 drops
Litsea Cubeba	5 drops
Pure Water	2 fl oz (60 ml)

Body-Scenting Mist

Rose	20 drops
Geranium	5 drops
Litsea Cubeba	5 drops
Sandalwood	5 drops
Pure Water	2 fl oz (60 ml)

Body-Scenting Mist

Champaca Flower	10 drops
Vanilla	10 drops
Lavender	10 drops
Bergamot	5 drops
Pure Water	2 fl oz (60 ml)

Body-Scenting Mist

Spruce	15 drops
Lavender	15 drops
Cedarwood (Atlas)	5 drops
Pure Water	2 fl oz (60 ml)

Body-Scenting Mist

Neroli	10 drops
Ylang-Ylang	10 drops
St.-John's-Wort	10 drops
Vanilla	5 drops
Pure Water	2 fl oz (60 ml)

Body-Scenting Mist

Rose	20 drops
Champaca Flower	5 drops
Pimento Berry	5 drops
Sandalwood	5 drops
Pure Water	2 fl oz (60 ml)

Body-Scenting Mist

Lavender	10 drops
Ylang-Ylang	10 drops
Labdanum (Cistus)	10 drops
Tangerine	5 drops
Pure Water	2 fl oz (60 ml)

BODY POWDERS

Select one of these formulas. Measure the amount of cornstarch and pour it into a small widemouthed glass jar or spice-powder container. Add the essential oils, mix thoroughly, then place the cap on the jar and tighten. Let the powder sit for a day so that the fragrance of the oils can permeate the powder.

Apply a small portion on the skin and rub in well. Store in a dark, cool place.

Helpful Measurement: 4 tablespoons (60 ml) of cornstarch weighs about 1 ounce or 28 grams.

Body Powder

Spearmint	25 drops
Vanilla	20 drops
Lavender	15 drops
Cornstarch	4 T (28 g)

Body Powder

Litsea Cubeba	35 drops
Vanilla	20 drops
Patchouli	5 drops
Cornstarch	4 T (28 g)

Body Powder

Lime	50 drops
Ylang-Ylang	10 drops
Cornstarch	4 T (28 g)

Body Powder

Neroli	25 drops
Tangerine	20 drops
Champaca Flower	15 drops
Cornstarch	4 T (28 g)

Body Powder

Ylang-Ylang	45 drops
Lemon	15 drops
Cornstarch	4 T (28 g)

Body Powder

Rose	45 drops
Orange	15 drops
Cornstarch	4 T (28 g)

PERFUMES

Select one of these formulas. Combine the vodka (80- to 100-proof), pure water, and jojoba in a glass perfume bottle with a fine-mist sprayer. Add the essential oils. Tighten the cap and shake well. Let the perfume age for about 30 days, periodically shaking the bottle to mix the oils. As the perfume continues to age, it will become stronger and nicer in fragramce. Store in a dark, cool place.

Perfume

Vanilla	60 drops
Cedarwood (Atlas)	60 drops
St.-John's-Wort	50 drops
Rose	45 drops
Lime	35 drops
Sandalwood	30 drops
Lavender	20 drops
Jojoba	2 t (10 ml)
Vodka	1 fl oz (30 ml)
Purified Water	1½ t (7.5 ml)

Perfume

Champaca Flower	90 drops
Rose	90 drops
Geranium	45 drops
Ylang-Ylang	30 drops
Orange	30 drops
Vanilla	15 drops
Jojoba	2 t (10 ml)
Vodka	1 fl oz (30 ml)
Purified Water	1½ t (7.5 ml)

Perfume

Cedarwood (Atlas)	60 drops
Lavender	60 drops
Spruce	60 drops
Lime	30 drops
Lemon	30 drops
Bergamot	30 drops
Sandalwood	20 drops
Clove Bud	10 drops
Jojoba	2 t (10 ml)
Vodka	1 fl oz (30 ml)
Purified Water	1½ t (7.5 ml)

PERSONAL CARE

BREATH FRESHENERS

Select one of these formulas. Fill a fine-mist-spray glass bottle with 2 fluid ounces (60 ml) of purified water, add the essential oils, tighten the cap, and shake well. Before using, shake again, and gently mist once or twice directly into the mouth. Enjoy the freshness! Store in a dark, cool place.

Breath Freshener

Peppermint	7 drops
Orange	3 drops
Pure Water	2 fl oz (60 ml)

Breath Freshener

Peppermint	7 drops
Anise	3 drops
Pure Water	2 fl oz (60 ml)

Breath Freshener

Helichrysum	4 drops
Cinnamon Bark	3 drops
Orange	3 drops
Pure Water	2 fl oz (60 ml)

Breath Freshener

Helichrysum	8 drops
Anise	2 drops
Pure Water	2 fl oz (60 ml)

Breath Freshener

Tangerine	4 drops
Clove Bud	3 drops
Sage (Spanish)	3 drops
Pure Water	2 fl oz (60 ml)

Breath Freshener

Spearmint	10 drops
Pure Water	2 fl oz (60 ml)

DEODORANTS & UNDERARM POWDERS

Select one of these formulas. Measure the amount of cornstarch and pour it into a small widemouthed glass jar, add the essential oils, and mix thoroughly. Tighten the cap and let the mixture sit for a day to allow the scent to permeate the powder.

Apply a small portion to the underarms and rub in well. Store in a dark, cool place.

Helpful Measurement: 4 tablespoons (60 ml) of cornstarch equals 1 ounce or 28 grams.

Deodorant & Underarm Powder

Manuka	55 drops
Vanilla	15 drops
Cornstarch	4 T (28 g)

Deodorant & Underarm Powder

Cabreuva	45 drops
Vanilla	15 drops
Niaouli	10 drops
Cornstarch	4 T (28 g)

SHOE & SNEAKER DEODORIZERS

Select one of these formulas. Using a glass dropper, apply the formula on two old cotton socks or cotton cloths. Fold the cloths over and make sure that the essential oils are on the inside of the cloth or sock. Then insert into the shoes or sneakers and let them sit. These deodorizers should leave your footwear smelling nice.

Shoe & Sneaker Deodorizer
Spearmint	24 drops
Cedarwood (Atlas)	6 drops

Shoe & Sneaker Deodorizer
Lemongrass	20 drops
Eucalyptus	6 drops
Copaiba	4 drops

Shoe & Sneaker Deodorizer

Clove Bud	20 drops
Orange	6 drops
Cedarwood (Atlas)	4 drops

Shoe & Sneaker Deodorizer

Peppermint	20 drops
Cassia Bark	6 drops
Lemon	4 drops

Shoe & Sneaker Deodorizer

Lemongrass	20 drops
Anise	10 drops

TOOTH POWDERS

Select one of these formulas. Measure the amount of arrowroot powder and pour it into a small wide-mouthed glass jar. Add the essential oils, stir well, and tighten the cap. Let the powder sit for a day.

Mix again before using, and brush your teeth with a small amount each time. Store in a dark, cool place.

Helpful Measurement: 4 tablespoons (60 ml) of arrowroot powder weighs about 1½ ounces or 42 grams.

Tooth Powder

Helichrysum	60 drops
Arrowroot Powder	4 T (42 g)

Tooth Powder

Spearmint	45 drops
Sage (Spanish)	15 drops
Arrowroot Powder	4 T (42 g)

BABY CARE

BABY'S BOTTOM CRÈMES

To help soothe and protect your baby's bottom between diaper changes, use a small amount of one of these formulas when changing the diaper.

Place the shea butter into a widemouthed glass jar and put the jar in a small cooking pot of water. Heat on low flame. When the shea butter has melted, add the sesame oil and stir well. Remove the jar from the heated water, and as the ingredients cool, mix in the essential oils well. Then place the cap on the jar and tighten. Let the crème sit for several hours until it becomes creamy in texture. Store in a dark, cool place.

Helpful Measurement: 2 tablespoons (30 ml) of shea butter weighs about 1 ounce or 28 grams.

Baby's Bottom Crème

Lavender	10 drops
Shea Butter	2 T (28 g)
Sesame Oil	8 t (40 ml)

Baby's Bottom Crème

Neroli	5 drops
Lavender	5 drops
Shea Butter	2 T (28 g)
Sesame Oil	8 t (40 ml)

Baby's Bottom Crème

Rose	5 drops
Lavender	5 drops
Shea Butter	2 T (28 g)
Sesame Oil	8 t (40 ml)

Baby's Bottom Crème

Tea Tree	5 drops
Lavender	5 drops
Shea Butter	2 T (28 g)
Sesame Oil	8 t (40 ml)

BABY'S BOTTOM POWDERS

To help keep your baby more comfortable, use a small amount of one of these formulas when changing the diaper.

Helpful Measurement: 2 tablespoons (30 ml) of cornstarch weighs about fi ounce or 14 grams.

Baby's Bottom Powder
Lavender	5 drops
Cornstarch	2 T (14 g)

Baby's Bottom Powder
Rose	3 drops
Lavender	2 drops
Cornstarch	2 T (14 g)

Baby's Bottom Powder
    Tea Tree   5 drops
    Cornstarch   2 T (14 g)

Baby's Bottom Powder
    Neroli   3 drops
    Lavender   2 drops
    Cornstarch   2 T (14 g)

CHAPTER 4

Inhalation for Mood & Effect

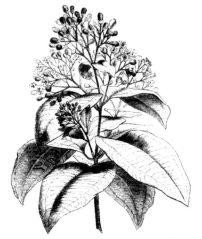

Cinnamon (*Cinnamomum verum*)

All of us have experienced memories triggered by specific aromas. The smell of pine and spruce trees may remind us of a place where we grew up during childhood; specific flowers may awaken memories of certain happy occasions we celebrated; or an aroma from a food may bring back fond thoughts of a particular person who prepared it.

Aromas affect us on a much deeper level than we realize, and they can influence our moods to a great extent.

AROMA LAMP

Select one of these formulas. Fill the small container on top of the aroma lamp with purified water, and add the essential oils. Depending on the type of aroma lamp you have, light the candle or turn on the lightbulb. As the water heats, the aromatic vapors diffuse into the air.

CHEER UP!

Cheer Up! (Aroma Lamp)

Peppermint	45 drops
Cinnamon Bark	3 drops
Eucalyptus	2 drops

Cheer Up! (Aroma Lamp)

Lemongrass	35 drops
Orange	10 drops
Ginger	5 drops

Cheer Up! (Aroma Lamp)

Lemongrass	27 drops
Tangerine	13 drops
Grapefruit	5 drops
Patchouli	5 drops

Cheer Up! (Aroma Lamp)

Lime	40 drops
Ylang-Ylang	10 drops

Cheer Up! (Aroma Lamp)

Spearmint	36 drops
Litsea Cubeba	9 drops
Vanilla	5 drops

Cheer Up! (Aroma Lamp)

Peppermint	35 drops
Frankincense	10 drops
Rosemary	5 drops

DIFFUSER

Select one of these formulas. Place the essential oils in the designated area of the diffuser, then turn on the unit to disperse the aroma into the air.

CALMING

Please avoid using these formulas prior to operating a motor vehicle or doing anything that requires full attention, since they may relax a person to the point where reflexes and other responses become slow.

Calming (Diffuser)

Chamomile	30%
Petitgrain	30%
Lemon	20%
Cinnamon Leaf	20%

Calming (Diffuser)
 Orange   50%
 Lemongrass   30%
 Juniper Berry   20%

Calming (Diffuser)
 Spruce   50%
 Lavender   50%

Calming (Diffuser)
 Mandarin   50%
 Lavender   50%

CHEER UP!

Cheer Up! (Diffuser)

Spearmint	50%
Lime	30%
Cinnamon Leaf	20%

Cheer Up! (Diffuser)

Spruce	40%
Peppermint	40%
Fir Needles	20%

Cheer Up! (Diffuser)

Litsea Cubeba	40%
Lime	40%
Tangerine	10%
Cinnamon Bark	10%

Cheer Up! (Diffuser)

Litsea Cubeba	50%
Bergamot	30%
Ylang-Ylang	20%

ENCOURAGE CONVERSATION

Encourage Conversation (Diffuser)

Spearmint	60%
Lemon	30%
Anise	10%

Encourage Conversation (Diffuser)

Grapefruit	50%
Tangerine	40%
Ginger	10%

Encourage Conversation (Diffuser)

Lime	50%
Litsea Cubeba	20%
Ylang-Ylang	20%
Clove Bud	10%

Encourage Conversation (Diffuser)

Peppermint	40%
Spearmint	40%
Basil (Sweet)	20%

MENTAL CLARITY

Mental Clarity (Diffuser)

Lime	50%
Spruce	50%

Mental Clarity (Diffuser)

Peppermint	90%
Cabreuva	10%

Mental Clarity (Diffuser)

Spearmint	70%
Tangerine	20%
Petitgrain	10%

Mental Clarity (Diffuser)

Lemongrass	50%
Lime	30%
Cinnamon Leaf	10%
Ravensara Aromatica	10%

REJUVENATING

Rejuvenating (Diffuser)

Spearmint	70%
Juniper Berry	20%
Cabreuva	10%

Rejuvenating (Diffuser)

Peppermint	60%
Fir Needles	20%
Clove Bud	20%

Rejuvenating (Diffuser)

Spearmint	80%
Clove Bud	20%

Rejuvenating (Diffuser)

Lime	50%
Lemongrass	30%
Cardamom	20%

RESTLESSNESS

Please avoid using these formulas prior to operating a motor vehicle or doing anything that requires full attention, since they may relax a person to the point where reflexes and other responses become slow.

Restlessness (Diffuser)

Petitgrain	50%
Mandarin	50%

Restlessness (Diffuser)

Mandarin	70%
Lavender	30%

Restlessness (Diffuser)

Mandarin	70%
Cypress	20%
Clary Sage	10%

Restlessness (Diffuser)

Orange	40%
Marjoram	40%
Pimento Berry	20%

INHALER

Inhalers are convenient to use, and they can provide beneficial results.

Select one of these formulas. Combine the essential oils in a small glass bottle with a wide opening. Tighten the cap and shake to mix the oils.

To use: Relax in a comfortable chair, uncap the bottle, and slowly inhale the vapors numerous times. Breathe deeply and avoid exhaling into the bottle. Immediately after using, cap the bottle and store in a dark, cool place. Use when needed.

Over a period of time, the inhaler may lose its potency as the vapors become faint. At that point, there is no need to discard the oils. Instead, combine them in a fine-mist-spray bottle with purified water, add fresh essential oils, and use as a mist spray.

BE MORE DECISIVE

Be More Decisive (Inhaler)

Peppermint	25 drops
Lime	15 drops
Cedarwood (Atlas)	10 drops

Be More Decisive (Inhaler)

Orange	20 drops
Cardamom	20 drops
Bergamot	10 drops

Be More Decisive (Inhaler)

Bergamot	20 drops
Spearmint	20 drops
Thyme	5 drops
Vetiver	5 drops

Be More Decisive (Inhaler)

Helichrysum	25 drops
Basil (Sweet)	15 drops
Bergamot	10 drops

Be More Decisive (Inhaler)

Helichrysum	20 drops
Grapefruit	20 drops
Thyme	10 drops

Be More Decisive (Inhaler)

Peppermint	25 drops
Basil (Sweet)	15 drops
Cabreuva	10 drops

CALMING

Please avoid using these formulas prior to operating a motor vehicle or doing anything that requires full attention, since they may relax a person to the point where reflexes and other responses become slow.

Calming (Inhaler)

Ylang-Ylang	20 drops
Lemon	20 drops
Petitgrain	10 drops

Calming (Inhaler)

Mandarin	20 drops
Rose	15 drops
Bergamot	10 drops
Pimento Berry	5 drops

Calming (Inhaler)

Tangerine	25 drops
Neroli	15 drops
Vetiver	10 drops

Calming (Inhaler)

Tangerine	20 drops
Chamomile	20 drops
Sandalwood	10 drops

Calming (Inhaler)

Frankincense	20 drops
Vanilla	20 drops
Mandarin	10 drops

Calming (Inhaler)

Vanilla	20 drops
Neroli	15 drops
Petitgrain	15 drops

CHEER UP!

Cheer Up! (Inhaler)

Orange	18 drops
Rose	15 drops
Lime	10 drops
Litsea Cubeba	7 drops

Cheer Up! (Inhaler)

Spruce	20 drops
Spearmint	20 drops
Cabreuva	10 drops

Cheer Up! (Inhaler)

Spearmint	25 drops
St.-John's-Wort	15 drops
Vanilla	10 drops

Cheer Up! (Inhaler)

Mandarin	15 drops
Bergamot	15 drops
Lemon	15 drops
Sage (Spanish)	5 drops

Cheer Up! (Inhaler)

Peppermint	20 drops
Gingergrass	15 drops
Lemongrass	15 drops

Cheer Up! (Inhaler)

Frankincense	30 drops
Vanilla	20 drops

ENCOURAGE CONVERSATION

Encourage Conversation (Inhaler)

Lemon	30 drops
Ylang-Ylang	15 drops
Clove Bud	5 drops

Encourage Conversation (Inhaler)

Vanilla	25 drops
Spruce	15 drops
Fir Needles	10 drops

Encourage Conversation (Inhaler)

Peppermint	40 drops
Havozo Bark	10 drops

Encourage Conversation (Inhaler)

Peppermint	20 drops
Lemongrass	20 drops
Gingergrass	10 drops

Encourage Conversation (Inhaler)

Frankincense	25 drops
Spearmint	25 drops

Encourage Conversation (Inhaler)

Tangerine	20 drops
Fir Needles	20 drops
Grapefruit	10 drops

MENTAL CLARITY

Mental Clarity (Inhaler)

Peppermint	20 drops
Tangerine	20 drops
Gingergrass	10 drops

Mental Clarity (Inhaler)

Ravensara Aromatica	20 drops
Lime	20 drops
Niaouli	10 drops

Mental Clarity (Inhaler)

Lemon	20 drops
Basil (Sweet)	15 drops
Bay (West Indian)	15 drops

Mental Clarity (Inhaler)

Juniper Berry	20 drops
Tangerine	20 drops
Lemongrass	10 drops

Mental Clarity (Inhaler)

Peppermint	25 drops
Eucalyptus	20 drops
Fir Needles	5 drops

Mental Clarity (Inhaler)

Lemongrass	30 drops
Rosemary	15 drops
Patchouli	5 drops

Mental Clarity (Inhaler)

Peppermint	35 drops
Neroli	15 drops

Mental Clarity (Inhaler)

Spearmint	35 drops
Petitgrain	10 drops
Cabreuva	5 drops

PMS EASE

PMS Ease (Inhaler)

Neroli	20 drops
Vanilla	15 drops
Petitgrain	10 drops
Fennel (Sweet)	5 drops

PMS Ease (Inhaler)

Mandarin	20 drops
Cypress	15 drops
Lavender	10 drops
Bergamot	5 drops

PMS Ease (Inhaler)

Mandarin	20 drops
Rose	15 drops
Lavender	15 drops

PMS Ease (Inhaler)

Helichrysum	20 drops
Mandarin	15 drops
Dill	15 drops

PMS Ease (Inhaler)

Neroli	20 drops
Vanilla	20 drops
Dill	10 drops

PMS Ease (Inhaler)

Mandarin	20 drops
Juniper Berry	10 drops
Vanilla	10 drops
Lemongrass	10 drops

PMS Ease (Inhaler)
  Rose   25 drops
  Sandalwood   15 drops
  Lime   10 drops

PMS Ease (Inhaler)
  Lemongrass   20 drops
  Rose   20 drops
  Neroli   10 drops

REJUVENATING

Rejuvenating (Inhaler)

Peppermint	45 drops
Patchouli	5 drops

Rejuvenating (Inhaler)

Lime	35 drops
Basil (Sweet)	10 drops
Black Pepper	5 drops

Rejuvenating (Inhaler)

Peppermint	43 drops
Sage (Spanish)	7 drops

Rejuvenating (Inhaler)

Lime	30 drops
Grapefruit	10 drops
Cardamom	10 drops

RESTLESSNESS

Please avoid using these formulas prior to operating a motor vehicle or doing anything that requires full attention, since they may relax a person to the point where reflexes and other responses become slow.

Restlessness (Inhaler)

Tangerine	30 drops
Ylang-Ylang	10 drops
Amyris	10 drops

Restlessness (Inhaler)

Spruce	25 drops
Petitgrain	15 drops
Chamomile	10 drops

Restlessness (Inhaler)

Mandarin	30 drops
Neroli	15 drops
Vetiver	5 drops

Restlessness (Inhaler)

Orange	20 drops
Rose	15 drops
Lemon	15 drops

Restlessness (Inhaler)

Vanilla	20 drops
Elemi	20 drops
Neroli	10 drops

Restlessness (Inhaler)

Mandarin	40 drops
Vetiver	10 drops

SLEEP RESTFULLY

Please avoid using these formulas prior to operating a motor vehicle or doing anything that requires full attention, since they may relax a person to the point where reflexes and other responses become slow.

Sleep Restfully (Inhaler)

Lavender	25 drops
Orange	15 drops
Elemi	10 drops

Sleep Restfully (Inhaler)

Vanilla	18 drops
Elemi	15 drops
Neroli	10 drops
Pimento Berry	7 drops

Sleep Restfully (Inhaler)

Mandarin	20 drops
Clary Sage	20 drops
Neroli	10 drops

Sleep Restfully (Inhaler)

Marjoram	25 drops
Amyris	15 drops
Elemi	10 drops

Sleep Restfully (Inhaler)

Vanilla	25 drops
Tangerine	15 drops
Spikenard	10 drops

Sleep Restfully (Inhaler)

Marjoram	20 drops
Celery	15 drops
Vanilla	10 drops
Cinnamon Leaf	5 drops

STIMULATE YOUR CREATIVE ABILITIES

Stimulate Your Creative Abilities (Inhaler)

Helichrysum	20 drops
Mandarin	20 drops
Basil (Sweet)	10 drops

Stimulate Your Creative Abilities (Inhaler)

Cinnamon Leaf	20 drops
Rose	20 drops
Hyssop Decumbens	10 drops

Stimulate Your Creative Abilities (Inhaler)

Helichrysum	15 drops
Spruce	15 drops
Lime	15 drops
Frankincense	5 drops

Stimulate Your Creative Abilities (Inhaler)

Tangerine	20 drops
Cinnamon Leaf	15 drops
Basil (Sweet)	15 drops

MIST SPRAYS

Select one of these formulas. Fill a fine-mist-spray glass bottle with 4 fluid ounces (120 ml) of purified water, add the essential oils, tighten the cap, and shake well. Before using, shake well again.

Sit comfortably in a chair and position the mist sprayer about 1 foot (30 cm) directly over your head, facing toward the front so that the mist falls in front of the face. Close your eyes and spray approximately ten times over the head. Stop with every two to three sprays and inhale deeply. Avoid getting any spray in the eyes. If you do, flush with cool water.

Store in a dark, cool place.

BE MORE DECISIVE

Be More Decisive (Mist Spray)

Peppermint	70 drops
Orange	50 drops
Cedarwood (Atlas)	30 drops
Pure Water	4 fl oz (120 ml)

Be More Decisive (Mist Spray)

Lime	60 drops
Peppermint	50 drops
Patchouli	20 drops
Cedarwood (Atlas)	20 drops
Pure Water	4 fl oz (120 ml)

Be More Decisive (Mist Spray)

Bergamot	60 drops
Spearmint	60 drops
Thyme	20 drops
Vetiver	10 drops
Pure Water	4 fl oz (120 ml)

Be More Decisive (Mist Spray)

Lime	75 drops
Sandalwood	25 drops
Cedarwood (Atlas)	25 drops
Rosemary	25 drops
Pure Water	4 fl oz (120 ml)

Be More Decisive (Mist Spray)

Peppermint	75 drops
Cabreuva	25 drops
Basil (Sweet)	25 drops
Lemon	25 drops
Pure Water	4 fl oz (120 ml)

Be More Decisive (Mist Spray)

Helichrysum	50 drops
Litsea Cubeba	50 drops
Lime	25 drops
Thyme	25 drops
Pure Water	4 fl oz (120 ml)

Be More Decisive (Mist Spray)

Bergamot	50 drops
Helichrysum	50 drops
Basil (Sweet)	30 drops
Cypress	20 drops
Pure Water	4 fl oz (120 ml)

Be More Decisive (Mist Spray)

Lemon	40 drops
Sandalwood	30 drops
Rose	30 drops
Cedarwood (Atlas)	30 drops
Black Pepper	20 drops
Pure Water	4 fl oz (120 ml)

CALMING

Please avoid using these formulas prior to operating a motor vehicle or doing anything that requires full attention, since they may relax a person to the point where reflexes and other responses become slow.

Calming (Mist Spray)

Orange	50 drops
Lavender	40 drops
Chamomile	20 drops
Petitgrain	20 drops
Sandalwood	20 drops
Pure Water	4 fl oz (120 ml)

Calming (Mist Spray)

Marjoram	50 drops
Vanilla	40 drops
Ylang-Ylang	30 drops
Elemi	30 drops
Pure Water	4 fl oz (120 ml)

Calming (Mist Spray)

Orange	60 drops
Neroli	50 drops
Petitgrain	20 drops
Cypress	10 drops
Vetiver	10 drops
Pure Water	4 fl oz (120 ml)

Calming (Mist Spray)

Mandarin	70 drops
Neroli	30 drops
Petitgrain	25 drops
Vanilla	20 drops
Vetiver	5 drops
Pure Water	4 fl oz (120 ml)

Calming (Mist Spray)
 Mandarin 70 drops
 Rose 40 drops
 Lime 20 drops
 Clove Bud 10 drops
 Guaiacwood 10 drops
 Pure Water 4 fl oz (120 ml)

Calming (Mist Spray)
 Lemongrass 80 drops
 Spikenard 40 drops
 Vanilla 30 drops
 Pure Water 4 fl oz (120 ml)

CHEER UP!

Cheer Up! (Mist Spray)

Grapefruit	40 drops
Orange	40 drops
Lime	40 drops
Rose	30 drops
Pure Water	4 fl oz (120 ml)

Cheer Up! (Mist Spray)

Peppermint	60 drops
Spruce	40 drops
Cabreuva	30 drops
Basil (Sweet)	20 drops
Pure Water	4 fl oz (120 ml)

Cheer Up! (Mist Spray)

Peppermint	70 drops
Vanilla	40 drops
Lemongrass	40 drops
Pure Water	4 fl oz (120 ml)

Cheer Up! (Mist Spray)

Spearmint	75 drops
Bergamot	35 drops
Neroli	30 drops
Vetiver	10 drops
Pure Water	4 fl oz (120 ml)

Cheer Up! (Mist Spray)

Ylang-Ylang	60 drops
Lemon	50 drops
Vanilla	30 drops
Basil (Sweet)	10 drops
Pure Water	4 fl oz (120 ml)

Cheer Up! (Mist Spray)

Vanilla	50 drops
Spruce	40 drops
Niaouli	30 drops
Litsea Cubeba	30 drops
Pure Water	4 fl oz (120 ml)

ENCOURAGE CONVERSATION

Encourage Conversation (Mist Spray)

Ylang-Ylang	50 drops
Litsea Cubeba	50 drops
Lemon	30 drops
Clove Bud	20 drops
Pure Water	4 fl oz (120 ml)

Encourage Conversation (Mist Spray)

Peppermint	75 drops
Spruce	50 drops
Lemon	15 drops
Spearmint	10 drops
Pure Water	4 fl oz (120 ml)

Encourage Conversation (Mist Spray)

Peppermint	80 drops
Vanilla	40 drops
Fir Needles	30 drops
Pure Water	4 fl oz (120 ml)

Encourage Conversation (Mist Spray)

Frankincense	50 drops
Spearmint	50 drops
Lemongrass	25 drops
Gingergrass	25 drops
Pure Water	4 fl oz (120 ml)

Encourage Conversation (Mist Spray)

Bergamot	60 drops
Lemongrass	50 drops
Vanilla	25 drops
Geranium	15 drops
Pure Water	4 fl oz (120 ml)

Encourage Conversation (Mist Spray)

Lemongrass	55 drops
Grapefruit	40 drops
Havozo Bark	40 drops
Patchouli	15 drops
Pure Water	4 fl oz (120 ml)

MENTAL CLARITY

Mental Clarity (Mist Spray)

Peppermint	70 drops
Tangerine	35 drops
Gingergrass	25 drops
Cabreuva	20 drops
Pure Water	4 fl oz (120 ml)

Mental Clarity (Mist Spray)

Lemongrass	50 drops
Rosemary	40 drops
Niaouli	40 drops
Cedarwood (Atlas)	20 drops
Pure Water	4 fl oz (120 ml)

Mental Clarity (Mist Spray)

Cardamom	55 drops
Tangerine	50 drops
Lime	25 drops
Grapefruit	20 drops
Pure Water	4 fl oz (120 ml)

Mental Clarity (Mist Spray)

Lime	75 drops
Tangerine	40 drops
Bay (West Indian)	20 drops
Basil (Sweet)	15 drops
Pure Water	4 fl oz (120 ml)

Mental Clarity (Mist Spray)

Cajeput	40 drops
Ravensara Aromatica	40 drops
Litsea Cubeba	30 drops
Lemon	20 drops
Grapefruit	20 drops
Pure Water	4 fl oz (120 ml)

Mental Clarity (Mist Spray)

Mandarin	45 drops
Lemongrass	45 drops
Basil (Sweet)	35 drops
Cypress	25 drops
Pure Water	4 fl oz (120 ml)

Mental Clarity (Mist Spray)

Peppermint	50 drops
Spruce	50 drops
Eucalyptus	30 drops
Lime	20 drops
Pure Water	4 fl oz (120 ml)

Mental Clarity (Mist Spray)

Petitgrain	40 drops
Bergamot	40 drops
Helichrysum	40 drops
Peppermint	30 drops
Pure Water	4 fl oz (120 ml)

PMS EASE

PMS Ease (Mist Spray)

Orange	50 drops
Lemongrass	40 drops
Helichrysum	25 drops
Grapefruit	20 drops
Fennel (Sweet)	15 drops
Pure Water	4 fl oz (120 ml)

PMS Ease (Mist Spray)

Mandarin	70 drops
Cypress	40 drops
Frankincense	20 drops
Lime	20 drops
Pure Water	4 fl oz (120 ml)

PMS Ease (Mist Spray)

Lemongrass	70 drops
Dill	30 drops
Juniper Berry	30 drops
Helichyrsum	20 drops
Pure Water	4 fl oz (120 ml)

PMS Ease (Mist Spray)

Mandarin	50 drops
Dill	30 drops
Neroli	25 drops
Spearmint	25 drops
Lavender	20 drops
Pure Water	4 fl oz (120 ml)

PMS Ease (Mist Spray)

Bergamot	50 drops
Ylang-Ylang	50 drops
Ginger	25 drops
Vanilla	25 drops
Pure Water	4 fl oz (120 ml)

PMS Ease (Mist Spray)

Mandarin	60 drops
Helichrysum	45 drops
Lavender	25 drops
Rose	20 drops
Pure Water	4 fl oz (120 ml)

REJUVENATING

Rejuvenating (Mist Spray)

Peppermint	95 drops
Basil (Sweet)	25 drops
Spearmint	20 drops
Patchouli	10 drops
Pure Water	4 fl oz (120 ml)

Rejuvenating (Mist Spray)

Lime	80 drops
Grapefruit	45 drops
Cardamom	25 drops
Pure Water	4 fl oz (120 ml)

Rejuvenating (Mist Spray)

Peppermint	80 drops
Lime	40 drops
Sandalwood	30 drops
Pure Water	4 fl oz (120 ml)

Rejuvenating (Mist Spray)

Grapefruit	75 drops
Bergamot	40 drops
Cardamom	25 drops
Lemon	10 drops
Pure Water	4 fl oz (120 ml)

Rejuvenating (Mist Spray)

Spearmint	75 drops
Eucalyptus	40 drops
Litsea Cubeba	35 drops
Pure Water	4 fl oz (120 ml)

RESTLESSNESS

Please avoid using these formulas prior to operating a motor vehicle or doing anything that requires full attention, since they may relax a person to the point where reflexes and other responses become slow.

Restlessness (Mist Spray)

Mandarin	90 drops
Neroli	35 drops
Vetiver	25 drops
Pure Water	4 fl oz (120 ml)

Restlessness (Mist Spray)

Lavender	50 drops
Spruce	35 drops
Cinnamon Leaf	35 drops
Frankincense	30 drops
Pure Water	4 fl oz (120 ml)

Restlessness (Mist Spray)

Neroli	40 drops
Elemi	40 drops
Vanilla	40 drops
Amyris	30 drops
Pure Water	4 fl oz (120 ml)

Restlessness (Mist Spray)

Tangerine	80 drops
Vanilla	40 drops
Myrrh	30 drops
Pure Water	4 fl oz (120 ml)

Restlessness (Mist Spray)

Mandarin	65 drops
Rose	45 drops
Lemongrass	30 drops
Guaiacwood	10 drops
Pure Water	4 fl oz (120 ml)

Restlessness (Mist Spray)

Chamomile	60 drops
Cinnamon Leaf	35 drops
Tangerine	30 drops
Juniper Berry	25 drops
Pure Water	4 fl oz (120 ml)

SLEEP RESTFULLY

Please avoid using these formulas prior to operating a motor vehicle or doing anything that requires full attention, since they may relax a person to the point where reflexes and other responses become slow.

Sleep Restfully (Mist Spray)

Neroli	40 drops
Vanilla	40 drops
Dill	30 drops
Litsea Cubeba	20 drops
Pimento Berry	20 drops
Pure Water	4 fl oz (120 ml)

Sleep Restfully (Mist Spray)

Marjoram	50 drops
Elemi	40 drops
Amyris	25 drops
Celery	25 drops
Vanilla	10 drops
Pure Water	4 fl oz (120 ml)

Sleep Restfully (Mist Spray)

Mandarin	50 drops
Clary Sage	40 drops
Dill	20 drops
Lavender	20 drops
Spikenard	20 drops
Pure Water	4 fl oz (120 ml)

Sleep Restfully (Mist Spray)

Marjoram	60 drops
Petitgrain	30 drops
Havozo Bark	25 drops
Spruce	25 drops
Copaiba	10 drops
Pure Water	4 fl oz (120 ml)

Sleep Restfully (Mist Spray)

Orange	60 drops
Petitgrain	30 drops
Ylang-Ylang	20 drops
Spikenard	20 drops
Guaiacwood	20 drops
Pure Water	4 fl oz (120 ml)

Sleep Restfully (Mist Spray)

Chamomile	40 drops
Orange	40 drops
Marjoram	40 drops
Vanilla	30 drops
Pure Water	4 fl oz (120 ml)

Stimulate Your Creative Abilities

Stimulate Your Creative Abilities (Mist Spray)

Helichrysum	60 drops
Hyssop Decumbens	50 drops
Cinnamon Leaf	40 drops
Pure Water	4 fl oz (120 ml)

Stimulate Your Creative Abilities (Mist Spray)

Spruce	60 drops
Lemon	60 drops
Basil (Sweet)	30 drops
Pure Water	4 fl oz (120 ml)

Stimulate Your Creative Abilities (Mist Spray)

Tangerine	60 drops
Cinnamon Leaf	60 drops
Rose	30 drops
Pure Water	4 fl oz (120 ml)

Stimulate Your Creative Abilities (Mist Spray)

Mandarin	50 drops
Helichrysum	40 drops
Cinnamon Leaf	30 drops
Basil (Sweet)	30 drops
Pure Water	4 fl oz (120 ml)

CHAPTER 5

Massage Oil Blends

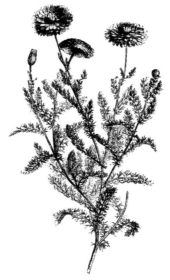

Roman Chamomile (*Anthemis nobilis*)

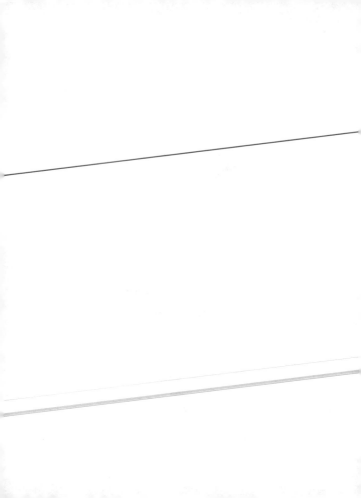

$\mathcal{M}$assage is the one of the oldest and most effective forms of therapy. Its healing power was well known in ancient times. Hippocrates, the father of medicine, in fourth century B.C. Greece, advocated that people receive a massage to maintain good health.

When essential oils are used on the skin, they need to be diluted with a carrier oil in order to prevent irritation. Where a carrier oil is specified in the massage-oil formulas, choose from the oils profiled in chapter 9, "Carrier Oil Profiles" (pp. 479–501).

AROMATHERAPY
MASGAGE TIPS

For best results when giving a massage, please follow these guidelines:

§ Wear comfortable clothing.

§ Fingernails should be short.

§ Use a massage table or place a firm cushion on the floor for the person receiving the massage.

§ Be in a calm and positive state of mind, since tension can easily be transferred to the receiver during the massage.

§ A room-fragrance formula can be used to create a nice scent in the room prior to the massage.

❧ Place all massage oils nearby to avoid searching for them during the massage.

❧ Wash hands with warm water before and after giving the massage.

❧ Warm the carrier oil by placing the bottle in warm water. Then pour an ample amount into the palm of your hand, rub both hands together, and then apply the oil on the receiver's skin.

❧ For best results, these formulas should be massaged into the skin for at least thirty minutes, until the oil is fully absorbed. Afterward, dry off the remaining oil on the skin by rubbing cornstarch on the area.

ACHES & PAINS

~

Massage one of these formulas into the specific and surrounding area(s) until the oil is fully absorbed into the skin.

Aches & Pains Massage Oil

Cabreuva	5 drops
Peppermint	4 drops
Oregano	3 drops
Manuka	3 drops
Carrier Oil	1 T (15 ml)

Aches & Pains Massage Oil

Marjoram	5 drops
Cinnamon Leaf	4 drops
Lavender	4 drops
Birch (Sweet)	2 drops
Carrier Oil	1 T (15 ml)

Aches & Pains Massage Oil

Ravensara Aromatica	4 drops
Caraway	4 drops
Peppermint	4 drops
Thyme	3 drops
Carrier Oil	1 T (15 ml)

Aches & Pains Massage Oil

Palmarosa	4 drops
St.-John's-Wort	4 drops
Spearmint	4 drops
Black Pepper	3 drops
Carrier Oil	1 T (15 ml)

Aches & Pains Massage Oil

Lemon	4 drops
Caraway	4 drops
Oregano	3 drops
Gingergrass	2 drops
Manuka	2 drops
Carrier Oil	1 T (15 ml)

Aches & Pains Massage Oil

Lavender	5 drops
Caraway	4 drops
Marjoram	3 drops
Cinnamon Leaf	3 drops
Carrier Oil	1 T (15 ml)

BE MORE DECISIVE

Massage one of these formulas into the back of the neck, upper chest, and shoulders until the oil is fully absorbed into the skin.

Be More Decisive Massage Oil

Spearmint	5 drops
Vetiver	5 drops
Thyme	3 drops
Cedarwood (Atlas)	2 drops
Carrier Oil	1 T (15 ml)

Be More Decisive Massage Oil

Helichrysum	5 drops
Orange	5 drops
Peppermint	5 drops
Carrier Oil	1 T (15 ml)

Be More Decisive Massage Oil

Cedarwood (Atlas)	5 drops
Thyme	4 drops
Sage (Spanish)	3 drops
Vetiver	3 drops
Carrier Oil	1 T (15 ml)

Be More Decisive Massage Oil

Black Pepper	4 drops
Grapefruit	4 drops
Orange	4 drops
Cedarwood (Atlas)	3 drops
Carrier Oil	1 T (15 ml)

Be More Decisive Massage Oil

Grapefruit	7 drops
Coriander	4 drops
Thyme	4 drops
Carrier Oil	1 T (15 ml)

Be More Decisive Massage Oil

Peppermint	5 drops
Basil (Sweet)	4 drops
Sage (Spanish)	4 drops
Orange	2 drops
Carrier Oil	1 T (15 ml)

BRIGHTEN YOUR OUTLOOK

~

At times, we feel overwhelmed by the complexities and pressures of modern life. Take some time out to contemplate on the direction of your life and what you can do to improve it.

Select one of these formulas. Find a comfortable, quiet place where you will not be disturbed. Have someone give you a massage or self-apply the massage blend on the back of your neck, upper chest, shoulders, and abdomen until the oil is fully absorbed into the skin. Then relax and open yourself up to allow thoughts and ideas to come to you on how to improve your life.

Do this massage and relaxation exercise a few times each week. In due time, you may surprise yourself with the ideas you can come up with to help you live a better life.

Brighten Your Outlook Massage Oil

Champaca Flower	5 drops
Frankincense	5 drops
Clary Sage	3 drops
Nutmeg	2 drops
Carrier Oil	1 T (15 ml)

Brighten Your Outlook Massage Oil

Cinnamon Leaf	4 drops
Rose	4 drops
Basil (Sweet)	4 drops
Guaiacwood	3 drops
Carrier Oil	1 T (15 ml)

Brighten Your Outlook Massage Oil

Clary Sage	3 drops
Chamomile	3 drops
Neroli	3 drops
Helichrysum	3 drops
Tangerine	3 drops
Carrier Oil	1 T (15 ml)

Brighten Your Outlook Massage Oil

St.-John's-Wort	5 drops
Helichrysum	4 drops
Vanilla	3 drops
Copaiba	3 drops
Carrier Oil	1 T (15 ml)

Brighten Your Outlook Massage Oil

Frankincense	4 drops
Neroli	4 drops
St.-John's-Wort	3 drops
Nutmeg	2 drops
Basil (Sweet)	2 drops
Carrier Oil	1 T (15 ml)

Brighten Your Outlook Massage Oil

Frankincense	4 drops
Bergamot	4 drops
Vanilla	3 drops
Grapefruit	2 drops
Basil (Sweet)	2 drops
Carrier Oil	1 T (15 ml)

Brighten Your Outlook Massage Oil

Neroli	4 drops
Copaiba	3 drops
Cinnamon Leaf	3 drops
Fennel (Sweet)	3 drops
Nutmeg	2 drops
Carrier Oil	1 T (15 ml)

CALMING

Massage one of these formulas into the back of the neck, shoulders, back, upper chest, and abdomen until the oil is fully absorbed into the skin.

Please avoid using these formulas prior to operating a motor vehicle or doing anything that requires full attention, since they may relax a person to the point where reflexes and other responses become slow.

Calming Massage Oil

Petitgrain	5 drops
Tangerine	5 drops
Myrrh	3 drops
Grapefruit	2 drops
Carrier Oil	1 T (15 ml)

Calming Massage Oil

Ylang-Ylang	5 drops
Sandalwood	5 drops
Neroli	5 drops
Carrier Oil	1 T (15 ml)

Calming Massage Oil

Neroli	5 drops
Cinnamon Leaf	4 drops
Frankincense	3 drops
Juniper Berry	3 drops
Carrier Oil	1 T (15 ml)

Calming Massage Oil

Litsea Cubeba	5 drops
Elemi	4 drops
Lavender	3 drops
Spruce	3 drops
Carrier Oil	1 T (15 ml)

Calming Massage Oil

Chamomile	3 drops
Neroli	3 drops
Rose	3 drops
Mandarin	3 drops
Sandalwood	3 drops
Carrier Oil	1 T (15 ml)

Calming Massage Oil

Dill	4 drops
Amyris	4 drops
Orange	4 drops
Cinnamon Leaf	3 drops
Carrier Oil	1 T (15 ml)

CHEER UP!

Massage one of these formulas into the back of the neck, shoulders, back, and upper chest until the oil is fully absorbed into the skin.

Cheer Up! Massage Oil

Spearmint	5 drops
Vanilla	5 drops
Lime	5 drops
Carrier Oil	1 T (15 ml)

Cheer Up! Massage Oil

Lemongrass	5 drops
Vanilla	5 drops
Sandalwood	5 drops
Carrier Oil	1 T (15 ml)

Cheer Up! Massage Oil

Lime	6 drops
Rose	4 drops
Clove Bud	3 drops
Tangerine	2 drops
Carrier Oil	1 T (15 ml)

Cheer Up! Massage Oil

Ylang-Ylang	5 drops
Neroli	4 drops
Mandarin	3 drops
Basil (Sweet)	3 drops
Carrier Oil	1 T (15 ml)

ENCOURAGE CONVERSATION

∾

Massage one of these formulas into the back of the neck, shoulders, and upper chest until the oil is fully absorbed into the skin.

Encourage Conversation Massage Oil

Vanilla	4 drops
Lemon	4 drops
Labdanum (Cistus)	4 drops
Orange	3 drops
Carrier Oil	1 T (15 ml)

Encourage Conversation Massage Oil

Frankincense	4 drops
Spruce	4 drops
Grapefruit	4 drops
Spearmint	3 drops
Carrier Oil	1 T (15 ml)

Encourage Conversation Massage Oil

Lemongrass	5 drops
Peppermint	5 drops
Geranium	3 drops
Tangerine	2 drops
Carrier Oil	1 T (15 ml)

Encourage Conversation Massage Oil

Lime	5 drops
Ylang-Ylang	4 drops
Basil (Sweet)	4 drops
Cabreuva	2 drops
Carrier Oil	1 T (15 ml)

Encourage Conversation Massage Oil

Spruce	5 drops
Peppermint	4 drops
St.-John's-Wort	3 drops
Anise	3 drops
Carrier Oil	1 T (15 ml)

Encourage Conversation Massage Oil

Fir Needles	5 drops
Spearmint	5 drops
Anise	3 drops
Geranium	2 drops
Carrier Oil	1 T (15 ml)

FEET & CALVES REFRESHERS
∾

These formulas soothe tired feet and can also be helpful when used prior to hiking or taking a long walk.

Select one of these formulas. Fill a basin with warm water and soak the feet for 10 minutes; then wipe dry. Massage the formula into the bottoms of the feet and up the calves until the oil is fully absorbed into the skin.

Feet & Calves Refresher Massage Oil

Helichrysum	5 drops
Geranium	4 drops
Rose	4 drops
Copaiba	2 drops
Carrier Oil	1 T (15 ml)

Feet & Calves Refresher Massage Oil

Spearmint	4 drops
Copaiba	4 drops
Oregano	3 drops
Geranium	2 drops
Gingergrass	2 drops
Carrier Oil	1 T (15 ml)

Feet & Calves Refresher Massage Oil

Cabreuva	5 drops
Helichrysum	5 drops
Peppermint	5 drops
Carrier Oil	1 T (15 ml)

Feet & Calves Refresher Massage Oil

Helichrysum	5 drops
Champaca Flower	5 drops
Rose	3 drops
Copaiba	2 drops
Carrier Oil	1 T (15 ml)

Feet & Calves Refresher Massage Oil

Ravensara Aromatica	4 drops
Spruce	4 drops
Spearmint	4 drops
Cajeput	3 drops
Carrier Oil	1 T (15 ml)

Feet & Calves Refresher Massage Oil

Lemongrass	6 drops
Black Pepper	3 drops
Patchouli	3 drops
Geranium	3 drops
Carrier Oil	1 T (15 ml)

GET CLOSER TO SOMONE
YOU CARE ABOUT

Giving a family member or friend a massage can play a great role in bringing people closer together. Find a comfortable quiet place, play soft music, and dim the lights. Massage one of these formulas into the back, shoulders, and upper chest until the oil is fully absorbed into the skin.

Get-Closer-to-Someone-You-Care-About Massage Oil

Mandarin	4 drops
Vanilla	4 drops
Anise	3 drops
Spearmint	2 drops
Petitgrain	2 drops
Carrier Oil	1 T (15 ml)

Get-Closer-to-Someone-You-Care-About Massage Oil

Sandalwood	3 drops
Vanilla	3 drops
Manuka	3 drops
Havozo Bark	3 drops
Cinnamon Leaf	3 drops
Carrier Oil	1 T (15 ml)

Get-Closer-to-Someone-You-Care-About Massage Oil

Neroli	5 drops
Mandarin	5 drops
Frankincense	5 drops
Carrier Oil	1 T (15 ml)

Get-Closer-to-Someone-You-Care-About Massage Oil

Neroli	5 drops
Manuka	3 drops
Orange	3 drops
Spearmint	2 drops
Clove Bud	2 drops
Carrier Oil	1 T (15 ml)

Get-Closer-to-Someone-You-Care-About Massage Oil

Champaca Flower	5 drops
Sandalwood	5 drops
Clove Bud	3 drops
Clary Sage	2 drops
Carrier Oil	1 T (15 ml)

Get-Closer-to-Someone-You-Care-About Massage Oil

Sandalwood	4 drops
Frankincense	4 drops
Tangerine	3 drops
Basil (Sweet)	2 drops
Spearmint	2 drops
Carrier Oil	1 T (15 ml)

HEAVENLY

Use these heavenly massage oil blends to elevate the mood and promote a state of greater well-being. Massage one of these formulas into the back, back of the neck, upper chest, shoulders, and abdomen until the oil is fully absorbed into the skin.

Heavenly Massage Oil

Sandalwood	4 drops
Frankincense	4 drops
Vanilla	4 drops
Tangerine	3 drops
Carrier Oil	1 T (15 ml)

Heavenly Massage Oil

Rose	5 drops
Bergamot	4 drops
Geranium	3 drops
Orange	3 drops
Carrier Oil	1 T (15 ml)

Heavenly Massage Oil

Litsea Cubeba	5 drops
Neroli	4 drops
Tangerine	4 drops
Spearmint	2 drops
Carrier Oil	1 T (15 ml)

Heavenly Massage Oil

Lemongrass	5 drops
Grapefruit	4 drops
Neroli	4 drops
Ginger	2 drops
Carrier Oil	1 T (15 ml)

Heavenly Massage Oil

Peppermint	4 drops
Vanilla	4 drops
Cabreuva	3 drops
Birch (Sweet)	2 drops
Grapefruit	2 drops
Carrier Oil	1 T (15 ml)

Heavenly Massage Oil

Ylang-Ylang	4 drops
Tangerine	4 drops
Lemongrass	4 drops
Vetiver	3 drops
Carrier Oil	1 T (15 ml)

Heavenly Massage Oil

Mandarin	5 drops
Tangerine	4 drops
Champaca Flower	3 drops
Cypress	3 drops
Carrier Oil	1 T (15 ml)

Heavenly Massage Oil

Frankincense	5 drops
Mandarin	5 drops
Grapefruit	5 drops
Carrier Oil	1 T (15 ml)

Heavenly Massage Oil

Champaca Flower	4 drops
Neroli	4 drops
Litsea Cubeba	4 drops
Amyris	2 drops
Orange	1 drop
Carrier Oil	1 T (15 ml)

Heavenly Massage Oil

Palmarosa	4 drops
Rose	4 drops
Vanilla	4 drops
Pimento Berry	3 drops
Carrier Oil	1 T (ml)

Heavenly Massage Oil

St.-John's-Wort	4 drops
Neroli	4 drops
Lemongrass	4 drops
Ylang-Ylang	3 drops
Carrier Oil	1 T (15 ml)

Heavenly Massage Oil

Lemon	5 drops
Frankincense	4 drops
St.-John's-Wort	4 drops
Chamomile	2 drops
Carrier Oil	1 T (15 ml)

IMPROVE PHYSICAL ENDURANCE

~

Perform an exercise, like sit-ups or push-ups, and record the number of repetitions you've achieved. Select one of these formulas and use it once a day for seven days. Massage the blend into the upper chest and the muscles that will be exerted until the oil is fully absorbed into the skin. Perform the same exercise each day after the massage, and compare your results on the seventh day with the number of repetitions initially recorded.

Improve Physical Endurance Massage Oil

Helichrysum	5 drops
Cabreuva	5 drops
Peppermint	5 drops
Carrier Oil	1 T (15 ml)

Improve Physical Endurance Massage Oil

Helichrysum	6 drops
Rose	5 drops
Manuka	4 drops
Carrier Oil	1 T (15 ml)

Improve Physical Endurance Massage Oil

Rose	6 drops
Thyme	5 drops
Copaiba	4 drops
Carrier Oil	1 T (15 ml)

Improve Physical Endurance Massage Oil

Rose	6 drops
Cabreuva	3 drops
Peppermint	3 drops
Oregano	3 drops
Carrier Oil	1 T (15 ml)

LOOSEN TIGHT MUSCLES
∿

Massage one of these formulas into tight muscles and the surrounding areas until the oil is fully absorbed into the skin.

Loosen Tight Muscles Massage Oil

Chamomile	4 drops
Lavender	4 drops
Vetiver	4 drops
Copaiba	3 drops
Carrier Oil	1 T (15 ml)

Loosen Tight Muscles Massage Oil

Labdanum (Cistus)	3 drops
Pimento Berry	3 drops
Cabreuva	3 drops
Rosemary	3 drops
Cinnamon Leaf	3 drops
Carrier Oil	1 T (15 ml)

Loosen Tight Muscles Massage Oil

Amyris	5 drops
Eucalyptus Radiata	4 drops
Bay (West Indian)	3 drops
Marjoram	3 drops
Carrier Oil	1 T (15 ml)

Loosen Tight Muscles Massage Oil

Cabreuva	4 drops
Elemi	4 drops
Oregano	4 drops
Manuka	3 drops
Carrier Oil	1 T (15 ml)

Loosen Tight Muscles Massage Oil

Niaouli	5 drops
Lavender	4 drops
Black Pepper	3 drops
Spruce	3 drops
Carrier Oil	1 T (15 ml)

Loosen Tight Muscles Massage Oil

Spikenard	5 drops
Cajeput	4 drops
Tangerine	4 drops
Cinnamon Leaf	2 drops
Carrier Oil	1 T (15 ml)

MENTAL CLARITY

༄

Massage one of these formulas into the back of the neck, shoulders, and upper chest until the oil is fully absorbed into the skin.

Mental Clarity Massage Oil

Mandarin	5 drops
Grapefruit	5 drops
Eucalyptus Radiata	3 drops
Cabreuva	2 drops
Carrier Oil	1 T (15 ml)

Mental Clarity Massage Oil

Lime	4 drops
Rosemary	4 drops
Copaiba	4 drops
Spearmint	3 drops
Carrier Oil	1 T (15 ml)

Mental Clarity Massage Oil

Tangerine	5 drops
Peppermint	4 drops
Lime	3 drops
Thyme	3 drops
Carrier Oil	1 T (15 ml)

Mental Clarity Massage Oil

Litsea Cubeba	5 drops
Eucalyptus Radiata	5 drops
Basil (Sweet)	3 drops
Cinnamon Leaf	2 drops
Carrier Oil	1 T (15 ml)

Mental Clarity Massage Oil

Lemongrass	5 drops
Cedarwood (Atlas)	4 drops
Helichrysum	4 drops
Black Pepper	2 drops
Carrier Oil	1 T (15 ml)

Mental Clarity Massage Oil

Ravensara Aromatica	4 drops
Juniper Berry	4 drops
Spearmint	4 drops
Coriander	3 drops
Carrier Oil	1 T (15 ml)

PMS EASE

Massage one of these formulas into the back of the neck, upper chest, and abdominal area until the oil is fully absorbed into the skin. Breathe the vapors in deeply. For best results, repeat application twice daily until relief is attained.

PMS-Ease Massage Oil

Ravensara Aromatica	5 drops
Fennel (Sweet)	5 drops
Mandarin	5 drops
Sesame Oil	2 t (10 ml)
Borage *or*	
Evening Primrose Oil	1 t (5 ml)

PMS-Ease Massage Oil

Neroli	4 drops
Rose	4 drops
Orange	4 drops
Petitgrain	3 drops
Sesame Oil	2 t (10 ml)
Borage *or*	
Evening Primrose Oil	1 t (5 ml)

PMS-Ease Massage Oil

Neroli	4 drops
Dill	4 drops
Mandarin	4 drops
Spearmint	3 drops
Sesame Oil	2 t (10 ml)
Borage *or*	
Evening Primrose Oil	1 t (5 ml)

PMS-Ease Massage Oil

Helichrysum	5 drops
Chamomile	5 drops
Juniper Berry	3 drops
Lavender	2 drops
Sesame Oil	2 t (10 ml)
Borage *or*	
Evening Primrose Oil	1 t (5 ml)

PMS-Ease Massage Oil

Lemongrass	4 drops
Chamomile	4 drops
Vanilla	4 drops
Neroli	3 drops
Sesame Oil	2 t (10 ml)
Borage *or*	
Evening Primrose Oil	1 t (5 ml)

PMS-Ease Massage Oil

Mandarin	4 drops
Fennel (Sweet)	4 drops
Cypress	3 drops
Petitgrain	2 drops
Ylang-Ylang	2 drops
Sesame Oil	2 t (10 ml)
Borage *or*	
Evening Primrose Oil	1 t (5 ml)

PRE-SPORTS

Use these pre-sports massage-oil blends to prepare the muscles to be more limber so that an athlete can perform better during sports competition. Massage one of these formulas into the shoulders, back, and leg muscles until the oil is fully absorbed into the skin.

Pre-Sports Massage Oil

Helichrysum	5 drops
Cabreuva	4 drops
Thyme	2 drops
Manuka	2 drops
Vanilla	2 drops
Carrier Oil	1 T (15 ml)

Pre-Sports Massage Oil

Peppermint	4 drops
Cabreuva	4 drops
Helichrysum	4 drops
Black Pepper	3 drops
Carrier Oil	1 T (15 ml)

Pre-Sports Massage Oil

Spearmint	5 drops
Copaiba	5 drops
Cajeput	3 drops
Oregano	2 drops
Carrier Oil	1 T (15 ml)

Pre-Sports Massage Oil

Helichrysum	5 drops
Ravensara Aromatica	3 drops
Eucalyptus	3 drops
Vanilla	2 drops
Spearmint	2 drops
Carrier Oil	1 T (15 ml)

RAINY-DAY COMFORT

To help brighten the mood on a rainy day, massage one of these formulas into the upper chest, neck, shoulders, and back until the oil is fully absorbed into the skin.

Rainy-Day-Comfort Massage Oil

Orange	6 drops
Cinnamon Leaf	4 drops
Juniper Berry	3 drops
Patchouli	2 drops
Carrier Oil	1 T (15 ml)

Rainy-Day-Comfort Massage Oil

Spearmint	5 drops
Cinnamon Leaf	4 drops
Anise	3 drops
Eucalyptus	3 drops
Carrier Oil	1 T (15 ml)

Rainy-Day-Comfort Massage Oil

Tangerine	7 drops
Cypress	4 drops
Thyme	4 drops
Carrier Oil	1 T (15 ml)

Rainy-Day-Comfort Massage Oil

Mandarin	5 drops
Helichrysum	4 drops
St.-John's-Wort	3 drops
Litsea Cubeba	3 drops
Carrier Oil	1 T (15 ml)

Rainy-Day-Comfort Massage Oil

Bergamot	5 drops
Rose	4 drops
Clove Bud	3 drops
Helichrysum	3 drops
Carrier Oil	1 T (15 ml)

Rainy-Day-Comfort Massage Oil

Lemongrass	5 drops
Juniper Berry	4 drops
Basil (Sweet)	3 drops
Geranium	3 drops
Carrier Oil	1 T (15 ml)

Rainy-Day-Comfort Massage Oil

St.-John's-Wort	4 drops
Vanilla	3 drops
Sandalwood	3 drops
Lemongrass	3 drops
Ylang-Ylang	2 drops
Carrier Oil	1 T (15 ml)

REJUVENATING

⌒

Massage one of these formulas into the back, neck, shoulders, and upper chest until the oil is fully absorbed into the skin.

Rejuvenating Massage Oil

Helichrysum	6 drops
Cardamom	5 drops
Grapefruit	4 drops
Carrier Oil	1 T (15 ml)

Rejuvenating Massage Oil

Lemon	5 drops
Rosemary	5 drops
Peppermint	5 drops
Carrier Oil	1 T (15 ml)

Rejuvenating Massage Oil

Peppermint	6 drops
Petitgrain	6 drops
Black Pepper	3 drops
Carrier Oil	1 T (15 ml)

Rejuvenating Massage Oil

Spearmint	6 drops
Petitgrain	5 drops
Cinnamon Leaf	4 drops
Carrier Oil	1 T (15 ml)

RESTLESSNESS

~

Massage one of these formulas into the back, neck, shoulders, upper chest, and abdominal area until the oil is fully absorbed into the skin.

Please avoid using these formulas prior to operating a motor vehicle or doing anything that requires full attention, since they may relax a person to the point where reflexes and other responses become slow.

Restlessness Massage Oil

Tangerine	4 drops
St.-John's-Wort	4 drops
Vetiver	4 drops
Marjoram	3 drops
Carrier Oil	1 T (15 ml)

Restlessness Massage Oil

Mandarin	6 drops
Petitgrain	5 drops
Dill	4 drops
Carrier Oil	1 T (15 ml)

Restlessness Massage Oil

Neroli	6 drops
Amyris	5 drops
Oregano	4 drops
Carrier Oil	1 T (15 ml)

Restlessness Massage Oil

Guaiacwood	5 drops
Neroli	4 drops
Dill	3 drops
St.-John's-Wort	3 drops
Carrier Oil	1 T (15 ml)

SLEEP RESTFULLY

~

Massage one of these formulas into the back, neck, shoulders, and upper chest until the oil is fully absorbed into the skin.

Please avoid using these formulas prior to operating a motor vehicle or doing anything that requires full attention, since they may relax a person to the point where reflexes and other responses become slow.

Sleep Restfully Massage Oil

Vanilla	5 drops
Elemi	5 drops
Lavender	3 drops
Celery	2 drops
Carrier Oil	1 T (15 ml)

Sleep Restfully Massage Oil

Marjoram	5 drops
Amyris	5 drops
Mandarin	5 drops
Carrier Oil	1 T (15 ml)

Sleep Restfully Massage Oil

Dill	5 drops
Tangerine	4 drops
Lavender	4 drops
Vetiver	2 drops
Carrier Oil	1 T (15 ml)

Sleep Restfully Massage Oil

Spikenard	5 drops
Neroli	4 drops
Mandarin	3 drops
Oregano	3 drops
Carrier Oil	1 T (15 ml)

Sleep Restfully Massage Oil

Petitgrain	4 drops
Orange	4 drops
Lavender	4 drops
Vetiver	3 drops
Carrier Oil	1 T (15 ml)

Sleep Restfully Massage Oil

Mandarin	5 drops
Vanilla	4 drops
Celery	4 drops
Ylang-Ylang	2 drops
Carrier Oil	1 T (15 ml)

STIMULATE YOUR
CREATIVE ABILITIES

Massage one of these formulas into the back of the neck, shoulders, and upper chest until the oil is fully absorbed into the skin.

Stimulate Your Creative Abilities Massage Oil

Helichyrsum	5 drops
Hyssop Decumbens	5 drops
Mandarin	5 drops
Carrier Oil	1 T (15 ml)

Stimulate Your Creative Abilities Massage Oil

Helichrysum	4 drops
Lemon	4 drops
Lime	3 drops
Basil (Sweet)	3 drops
Carrier Oil	1 T (15 ml)

Stimulate Your Creative Abilities Massage Oil

Tangerine	5 drops
Spearmint	4 drops
Cinnamon Leaf	3 drops
Basil (Sweet)	3 drops
Carrier Oil	1 T (15 ml)

Stimulate Your Creative Abilities Massage Oil

Helichrysum	5 drops
Spruce	4 drops
Orange	4 drops
Black Pepper	3 drops
Carrier Oil	1 T (15 ml)

WARMING

Massage one of these formulas into the back of the neck, shoulders, back, upper chest, abdomen, hands, and feet until the oil is fully absorbed into the skin.

Warming Massage Oil

Fennel (Sweet)	4 drops
Cabreuva	4 drops
Cajeput	4 drops
Marjoram	3 drops
Carrier Oil	1 T (15 ml)

Warming Massage Oil

Havozo Bark	4 drops
Palmarosa	4 drops
Elemi	4 drops
Oregano	3 drops
Carrier Oil	1 T (15 ml)

Warming Massage Oil

Cabreuva	4 drops
Cardamom	4 drops
Elemi	4 drops
Champaca Flower	3 drops
Carrier Oil	1 T (15 ml)

Warming Massage Oil

Cajeput	4 drops
Palmarosa	4 drops
Marjoram	4 drops
Thyme	3 drops
Carrier Oil	1 T (15 ml)

CHAPTER 6

Home Products

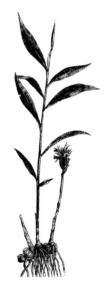

Ginger (*Zingiber officinale*)

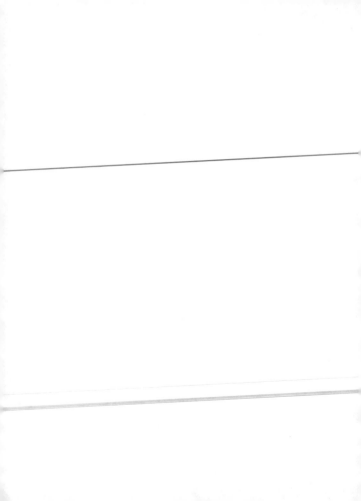

Today, it is commonplace for people to be exposed to thousands of chemicals daily—some very harmful to health. It is becoming more obvious to many people that we must take more responsibility for our actions and use products that are compatible with our natural environment.

Many plant essential oils can be combined to produce the finest, most effective formulas to improve the quality of life and, at the same time, be safe and nontoxic to our planet.

BATHROOM AIR FRESHENERS

Select one of these formulas. Fill a fine-mist-spray glass bottle with 4 fluid ounces (120 ml) of purified water. Add the essential oils, tighten the cap, and shake well. Mist numerous times in the room to freshen the air.

Bathroom Air Freshener (Mist Spray)

Peppermint	90 drops
Amyris	40 drops
Lavender	20 drops
Pure Water	4 fl oz (120 ml)

Bathroom Air Freshener (Mist Spray)

Orange	90 drops
Cinnamon Bark	30 drops
Copaiba	30 drops
Pure Water	4 fl oz (120 ml)

Bathroom Air Freshener (Mist Spray)

Lemongrass	55 drops
Orange	40 drops
Vetiver	30 drops
Lemon	20 drops
Ginger	5 drops
Pure Water	4 fl oz (120 ml)

Bathroom Air Freshener (Mist Spray)

Litsea Cubeba	95 drops
Grapefruit	30 drops
Patchouli	15 drops
Clove Bud	10 drops
Pure Water	4 fl oz (120 ml)

CARPET FRESHENERS

Select one of these formulas. Measure the bicarbonate of soda and pour it into a widemouthed glass jar, add the essential oils, and tighten the cap. Let the formula sit for a day to allow the scent to permeate the powder.

First test a small area of your carpet to make sure that there won't be any discoloration of the carpet fiber. Sprinkle over carpeting, leave for 10 to 15 minutes, and vacuum. Store the remainder of the powder in a dark, cool place.

Helpful Measurement: ½ cup or 8 tablespoons (120 ml) of bicarbonate of soda weighs about 5 ounces or about 142 grams.

Carpet Freshener

Spearmint	70 drops
Peppermint	40 drops
Lemon	20 drops
Copaiba	10 drops
Birch (Sweet)	10 drops
Bicarbonate of Soda	½ cup (142 g)

Carpet Freshener

Orange	50 drops
Lemongrass	50 drops
Grapefruit	30 drops
Clove Bud	20 drops
Bicarbonate of Soda	½ cup (142 g)

Carpet Freshener

Peppermint	80 drops
Spruce	50 drops
Fir Needle	20 drops
Bicarbonate of Soda	½ cup (142 g)

Carpet Freshener

Spearmint	50 drops
Tangerine	50 drops
Lavender	40 drops
Cassia Bark	10 drops
Bicarbonate of Soda	½ cup (142 g)

Carpet Freshener

Peppermint	70 drops
Spearmint	50 drops
Clove Bud	20 drops
Copaiba	10 drops
Bicarbonate of Soda	½ cup (142 g)

Carpet Freshener

Lime	60 drops
Litsea Cubeba	50 drops
Tangerine	30 drops
Ginger	10 drops
Bicarbonate of Soda	½ cup (142 g)

CABINET & FURNITURE POLISH
෴

Select one of these formulas. Place the shea butter into a widemouthed glass jar and put the jar in a small cooking pot of water. Heat on a low flame. When the butter has melted, add the jojoba oil and stir well. Then remove the jar from the heated water, and, as the ingredients cool, mix the essential oils in well. Place the cap on the jar and tighten. Let the polish sit for several hours until it thickens from its liquid state.

Before polishing, make sure the surface is clean. Then apply a small amount of polish on a soft cotton cloth. Gently rub the cloth over the surface of wooden cabinets and furniture until the wood has a nice shine. Store in a dark, cool place.

Helpful Measurement: 2 tablespoons (30 ml) of shea butter weighs about 1 ounce or about 28 grams.

Cabinet & Furniture Polish

Shea Butter	2 T (28 g)
Jojoba	1 t (5 ml)
Sandalwood	10 drops

Cabinet & Furniture Polish

Shea Butter	2 T (28 g)
Jojoba	1 t (5 ml)
Cedarwood (Atlas)	10 drops

Cabinet & Furniture Polish

Shea Butter	2 T (28 g)
Jojoba	1 t (5 ml)
Orange	5 drops
Ylang-Ylang	5 drops

PLANT SPRAYS FOR INSECTS

Insect problems can be handled in a nontoxic way using essential oils, which will also strengthen the plant. Use these plant sprays to repel insects before they begin to do harm.

Select one of these formulas. Fill a fine-mist-spray glass bottle with 4 fluid ounces (120 ml) of purified water. Add the essential oils and tighten the cap. Shake well and mist the plant. Use as small an amount as possible. Several applications, a few days apart, may be necessary.

Plant Spray for Insects

Lemongrass	40 drops
Lavender	40 drops
Rosemary	10 drops
Pure Water	4 fl oz (120 ml)

Plant Spray for Insects

Coriander	45 drops
Litsea Cubeba	40 drops
Copaiba	5 drops
Pure Water	4 fl oz (120 ml)

Plant Spray for Insects

Sage (Spanish)	40 drops
Lemongrass	40 drops
Black Pepper	10 drops
Pure Water	4 fl oz (120 ml)

Plant Spray for Insects

Sage (Spanish)	35 drops
Litsea Cubeba	30 drops
Cinnamon Leaf	25 drops
Pure Water	4 fl oz (120 ml)

Plant Spray for Insects

Lavender	40 drops
Coriander	25 drops
Copaiba	15 drops
Cinnamon Bark	10 drops
Pure Water	4 fl oz (120 ml)

Plant Spray for Insects

Cajeput	30 drops
Lavender	30 drops
Marjoram	20 drops
Copaiba	10 drops
Pure Water	4 fl oz (120 ml)

SANITIZERS FOR AWAY FROM HOME

When we come into contact with toilet seats, door knobs, and telephone receivers, we can easily pick up harmful strains of bacteria and viruses, especially during cold and flu season. These sanitizers can come in handy when traveling.

Select one of these formulas. Fill a fine-mist-spray glass bottle with 2 fluid ounces (60 ml) of purified water, add the essential oils, tighten the cap, and shake well.

To use: Shake well. Spray the mist on a cloth or tissue and wipe the area to be sanitized.

Sanitizer for Away from Home (Mist Spray)

Lavender	25 drops
Clove Bud	20 drops
Spearmint	20 drops
Patchouli	10 drops
Pure Water	2 fl oz (60 ml)

Sanitizer for Away from Home (Mist Spray)

Cinnamon Leaf	20 drops
Peppermint	20 drops
Eucalyptus	20 drops
Clove Bud	15 drops
Pure Water	2 fl oz (60 ml)

Sanitizer for Away from Home (Mist Spray)

Lemongrass	30 drops
Orange	30 drops
Pine	10 drops
Patchouli	5 drops
Pure Water	2 fl oz (60 ml)

Sanitizer for Away from Home (Mist Spray)

Lime	50 drops
Thyme	15 drops
Eucalyptus	10 drops
Pure Water	2 fl oz (60 ml)

Sanitizer for Away from Home (Mist Spray)

Peppermint	50 drops
Orange	20 drops
Birch (Sweet)	5 drops
Pure Water	2 fl oz (60 ml)

SANITIZERS FOR THE KITCHEN

After preparing food, clean the kitchen countertop and cutting board. Then spray one of these formulas several times over these areas and wipe dry.

Fill a fine-mist-spray glass bottle with 4 fluid ounces (120 ml) of purified water, add the essential oils, tighten the cap, and shake well.

To use: Shake well, spray over the area to be sanitized, and wipe dry with a cloth or paper towel.

Sanitizer for the Kitchen (Mist Spray)

Clove Bud	50 drops
Lavender	50 drops
Lemon	50 drops
Pure Water	4 fl oz (120 ml)

Sanitizer for the Kitchen (Mist Spray)

Lemongrass	60 drops
Orange	60 drops
Pine	20 drops
Patchouli	10 drops
Pure Water	4 fl oz (120 ml)

Sanitizer for the Kitchen (Mist Spray)

Peppermint	70 drops
Bay (West Indian)	30 drops
Orange	30 drops
Cinnamon Leaf	20 drops
Pure Water	4 fl oz (120 ml)

Sanitizer for the Kitchen (Mist Spray)

Lemon	50 drops
Grapefruit	40 drops
Lime	40 drops
Tea Tree	20 drops
Pure Water	4 fl oz (120 ml)

SANITIZERS FOR MATTRESSES

A mattress can harbor many undesirable organisms, like dust mites, bed bugs, lice, and all types of bacteria. These mist sprays are especially helpful when you are sleeping away from home in a hotel or motel.

Select one of these formulas. Fill a fine-mist-spray glass bottle with 2 fluid ounces (60 ml) of purified water, add the essential oils, tighten the cap, and shake well.

To use: Shake well. Spray the mattress several times in order to sanitize and freshen it. Then allow the mattress to air out for about an hour or two before putting the sheets and covers on.

Sanitizer for the Mattress (Mist Spray)

Peppermint	50 drops
Eucalyptus	10 drops
Oregano	10 drops
Pine	5 drops
Pure Water	2 fl oz (60 ml)

Sanitizer for the Mattress (Mist Spray)

Spearmint	50 drops
Thyme	15 drops
Lemon	10 drops
Pure Water	2 fl oz (60 ml)

Sanitizer for the Mattress (Mist Spray)

Peppermint	50 drops
Orange	22 drops
Cassia Bark	3 drops
Pure Water	2 fl oz (60 ml)

Sanitizer for the Mattress (Mist Spray)

Lavender	50 drops
Spearmint	20 drops
Marjoram	5 drops
Pure Water	2 fl oz (60 ml)

Sanitizer for the Mattress (Mist Spray)

Lavender	40 drops
Lemon	20 drops
Clove Bud	15 drops
Pure Water	2 fl oz (60 ml)

Sanitizer for the Mattress (Mist Spray)

Lemongrass	30 drops
Cinnamon Bark	25 drops
Oregano	20 drops
Pure Water	2 fl oz (60 ml)

Sanitizer for the Mattress (Mist Spray)

Lavender	40 drops
Manuka	20 drops
Copaiba	15 drops
Pure Water	2 fl oz (60 ml)

CHAPTER 7

Pet Care

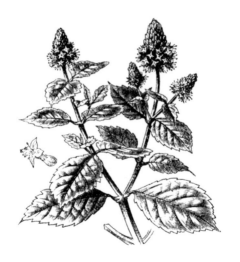

Patchouli (*Pogostemon patchouly*)

$\mathcal{P}$rotecting the family and home against crime, hauling sleds in the Arctic and Antarctica, and guiding the blind are some of the loyal duties dogs perform. The saying "A dog is a man's best friend" is certainly true.

Dogs, cats, and other animals present us with an important link to the natural world. Having a pet is a joy, but also a great responsibility.

When animals live in the wilderness, a close connection exists between themselves and their natural surroundings. Animals that are ill have been known to seek out and eat certain plants that are beneficial to them. But when domesticated animals are deprived of this opportunity, it becomes our responsibility to provide them with the best help we can in a natural way.

By using essential oils, we can create a better atmosphere for ourselves and our pets. So enjoy your loyal companions.

CALM A PET

In the wild, animals have vast areas in which to run, and they are able get more of their share of exercise. When domesticated, they may find it difficult acclimating to their new environment. Imagine how a person would feel being restricted to a designated area for long periods of time, or even chained to a post. It is important to allow an animal to run freely in an open field or forest area whenever possible.

If your animal is hyperactive, especially in the home, these calming formulas will help to calm the pet's nervous system.

MASSAGE OIL BLENDS

Select one of these formulas. Mix the oils together in a small glass bottle, and massage the formula into the tummy, the neck, and the back until the oil is absorbed into the skin. Then rub in cornstarch to dry any remaining oil from the fur.

Calm-a-Pet Massage Oil

Lavender	5 drops
Ylang-Ylang	4 drops
Sesame Oil	1 T (15 ml)

Calm-a-Pet Massage Oil

Marjoram	5 drops
Sandalwood	4 drops
Sesame Oil	1 T (15 ml)

Calm-a-Pet Massage Oil

Neroli	5 drops
Vetiver	3 drops
Vanilla	1 drop
Sesame Oil	1 T (15 ml)

Calm-a-Pet Massage Oil

Mandarin	3 drops
Spikenard	3 drops
Marjoram	3 drops
Sesame Oil	1 T (15 ml)

MIST SPRAYS

Select one of these formulas. Fill a fine-mist-spray glass bottle with 4 fluid ounces (120 ml) of purified water, add the essential oils, tighten the cap, and shake well.

To use: Shake well again and spray twice for every 10 pounds (4.5 kg) of body weight. Mist around the front of the animal. Avoid spraying directly into the animal's face.

Calm-a-Pet Mist Spray

Mandarin	40 drops
Vetiver	40 drops
Chamomile	40 drops
Pure Water	4 fl oz (120 ml)

Calm-a-Pet Mist Spray

Lavender	50 drops
Mandarin	50 drops
Amyris	20 drops
Pure Water	4 fl oz (120 ml)

Calm-a-Pet Mist Spray

Petitgrain	60 drops
Marjoram	60 drops
Pure Water	4 fl oz (120 ml)

Calm-a-Pet Mist Spray

Mandarin	40 drops
Copaiba	40 drops
Vetiver	25 drops
Anise	15 drops
Pure Water	4 fl oz (120 ml)

CUTS, BITES & IRRITATIONS

∾

Select one of these formulas. Wash the area with warm water, then apply aloe-vera juice or gel. Wait several minutes and then apply the formula to the affected area(s). Use as often as necessary.

Cuts, Bites & Irritations Soothing Oil

Lavender	3 drops
Sesame Oil	10 drops

Cuts, Bites & Irritations Soothing Oil

Tea Tree	3 drops
Sesame Oil	10 drops

DOGGY EAR-FLAP MIST SPRAYS

The area around a dog's ears seems to attract lots of pesty insects and bacteria. These formulas can help soothe the ears and relieve minor irritations.

Select one of these formulas. Fill a fine-mist-spray glass bottle with 4 fluid ounces (120 ml) of purified water, add the essential oils, tighten the cap, and shake well.

To use: Shake well. Gently spray around the dog's ears and inside the flap. Be careful not to get the mist near the dog's eyes.

Doggy Ear-Flap Mist Spray

Lavender	70 drops
Copaiba	30 drops
Manuka	20 drops
Pure Water	4 fl oz (120 ml)

Doggy Ear-Flap Mist Spray

Lavender	60 drops
Tea Tree	40 drops
Copaiba	20 drops
Pure Water	4 fl oz (120 ml)

Doggy Ear-Flap Mist Spray

Lavender	75 drops
Cajeput	35 drops
Manuka	10 drops
Pure Water	4 fl oz (120 ml)

Doggy Ear-Flap Mist Spray

Lavender	60 drops
Cedarwood (Atlas)	20 drops
Lemon	20 drops
Niaouli	20 drops
Pure Water	4 fl oz (120 ml)

Doggy Ear-Flap Mist Spray

Frankincense	40 drops
Manuka	30 drops
Ravensara Aromatica	30 drops
Cabreuva	20 drops
Pure Water	4 fl oz (120 ml)

Doggy Ear-Flap Mist Spray

Copaiba	40 drops
Sandalwood	20 drops
Chamomile	20 drops
Juniper Berry	20 drops
Pure Water	4 fl oz (120 ml)

Doggy Ear-Flap Mist Spray

Fir Needles	40 drops
Eucalyptus	30 drops
~~Lavender~~	~~30 drops~~
Pine	20 drops
Pure Water	4 fl oz (120 ml)

EAR ITCH

Before using, mix the oils well. Use a glass dropper, and drop the entire amount of the formula slowly into each ear. When dropping the oil into the dog's ear, make sure the animal is away from carpets and upholstery since the dog will tend to shake its head to try to remove the oil from the ear. Repeat for several days if needed.

Ear Itch Soothing Oil

Lavender	1 drop
Tea Tree	1 drop
Jojoba Oil	10 drops

STIFF JOINTS
~

Massage one of the formulas into the joint(s) until the oil is fully absorbed. Then rub on cornstarch to dry off the area.

Stiff Joints Massage Oil
    Lavender   4 drops
    Ginger   4 drops
    Sesame Oil   1 T (15 ml)

Stiff Joints Massage Oil
    Black Pepper   2 drops
    Manuka   2 drops
    Geranium   2 drops
    Copaiba   2 drops
    Sesame Oil   1 T (15 ml)

TICKS & FLEAS

∾

Tick & Flea Carpet Powder

Measure and pour the bicarbonate of soda into a widemouthed glass jar. Add the essential oils, stir well, and tightly cap the jar.

To use: First test a small area of your carpet to make sure that the formula will not discolor the carpet fiber. Sprinkle the powder over the carpet and leave it on as long as possible. Then vacuum. Store the powder in a dark, cool place.

Helpful Measurement: ½ cup or 8 tablespoons (120 ml) of bicarbonate of soda weighs about 5 ounces or 142 grams.

Tick & Flea Carpet Powder

Thyme	60 drops
Clove Bud	50 drops
Eucalyptus	20 drops
Litsea Cubeba	20 drops
Bicarbonate of Soda	½ cup (142 g)

TICK & FLEA MIST SPRAYS

Select one of these formulas. Fill a fine-mist-spray glass bottle with 4 fluid ounces (120 ml) of purified water, add the essential oils, tighten the cap, and shake well. To use: Spray the mist directly into the animal's coat and brush through the fur.

With each application of the mist, it is better to spray less than more, to make sure the animal does not get overly saturated with the oils. For best results, repeat regularly until the ticks and fleas are completely gone. Avoid getting the vapors near the animal's eyes, nose, and genital area.

In addition, use the tick and flea carpet powder (pp. 339–340) on floor areas where the pet stays.

Tick & Flea Mist Spray

Tea Tree	50 drops
Peppermint	50 drops
Copaiba	50 drops
Pure Water	4 fl oz (120 ml)

Tick & Flea Mist Spray

Lemongrass	50 drops
Lavender	40 drops
Cajeput	40 drops
Cedarwood (Atlas)	20 drops
Pure Water	4 fl oz (120 ml)

Tick & Flea Mist Spray

Peppermint	45 drops
Lavender	45 drops
Eucalyptus	40 drops
Lemongrass	10 drops
Patchouli	10 drops
Pure Water	4 fl oz (120 ml)

Tick & Flea Powders

Select one of the formulas. Measure and pour the cornstarch into a widemouthed glass jar, add the essential oils, stir well, and tightly cap the jar.

To use: First wash the animal with tick & flea preventative shampoo (pp. 345–346). When the fur is dry, brush or rub a portion of the powder into the coat. With each application, it is better to use less of the powder, rather than more, to make sure the animal does not get too saturated with the oils.

Apply as often as necessary. Avoid getting the powder near the animal's eyes, nose, and genitals. Use tick & flea carpet powder (pp. 339–340) on the carpeting as well as other floor areas where the insect eggs may exist.

Helpful Measurement: 8 tablespoons (120 ml) of cornstarch weighs about 2 ounces or 57 grams.

Tick & Flea Powder

Tea Tree	50 drops
Litsea Cubeba	50 drops
Patchouli	20 drops
Cornstarch	8 T (57 g)

Tick & Flea Powder

Cinnamon Leaf	50 drops
Rosemary	50 drops
Cedarwood (Atlas)	20 drops
Cornstarch	8 T (57 g)

TICK & FLEA PREVENTATIVE SHAMPOO

Shampoo your pet regularly to repel parasites and to keep the pet's coat clean.

Purchase the shampoo from your health-food store. Be certain it only contains natural ingredients. Combine the essential oils with 8 fluid ounces (240 ml) of the shampoo and shake well before using. Use a small amount of the shampoo each time.

Bathe your pet more frequently during the summer months, when ticks and fleas are most prevalent.

Tick & Flea Preventative Shampoo

Natural Shampoo	8 fl oz (240 ml)
Lemongrass	45 drops
Lavender	20 drops
Patchouli	10 drops

Tick & Flea Preventative Shampoo

Natural Shampoo	8 fl oz (240 ml)
Litsea Cubeba	45 drops
Tea Tree	20 drops
Cedarwood (Atlas)	10 drops

CHAPTER 8

Essential Oil Profiles

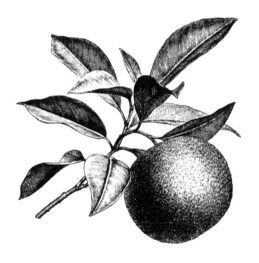

Orange (*Citrus sinensis*)

$\mathcal{E}$ssential oils are the precious essences extracted from herbs, flowers, and trees. These wonderful, pure, and fragrant oils contain a natural living substance known as the "essence," which is the concentrated power and vital life force of the plant. Every day we are presented with a great opportunity to enhance our environment and well-being with these remarkable essential oils. It is truly amazing the multitude of benefits and uses each individual oil offers us! In this chapter, over 70 essential oils are profiled to help you become more acquainted with the plants themselves and their valuable properties.

Please also refer to all safety guidelines in chapter 1, "Safe Use, Handling & Purity of Oils," (pp. 27–41).

AMYRIS

BOTANICAL NAME: *Amyris balsamifera*
FAMILY: Rutaceae

The Plant: Amyris is an evergreen tree native to the West Indies and Central America. The tree grows to about 60 feet (18 m) high and has clusters of white flowers that develop into edible bluish-black fruit. Also known as West Indian sandalwood, amyris should not be confused with true sandalwood.

The Essential Oil: The oil is extracted from the wood chips of the tree.

Scent of the Oil: Sweet, woody, smoky.

Main Uses

Calming; reduces stress, anxiety, and tension; promotes a peaceful state and restful sleep; quiets the mind; loosens tight muscles; used as a fixative to hold the scent of a fragrance.

Other Uses

Deepens breathing; mood uplifting; reviving; improves mental clarity.

ANISE

BOTANICAL NAME: *Pimpinella anisum*
FAMILY: *Apiaceae*
The Plant: Anise is native to the Mediterranean. The plant grows to about 2 feet (60 cm) high and has small white flowers.
The Essential Oil: The oil is extracted from the seeds of the plant.
Scent of the Oil: Warm, sweet, licoricelike.

Main Uses

Improves digestion; soothes the intestines; relieves flatulence and aerophagia; mood uplifting; improves communication; lessens pain; helps ease menstrual discomfort.

Other Uses

Warming; calming; relaxing; promotes restful

sleep; vapors open sinuses and breathing passages; increases lactation.

Precautions: People with dry or sensitive skin may require additional carrier oil when using anise essential oil on the skin. Anise tends to slow down reflexes. Avoid driving or doing anything that requires full attention after using the oil. Use small amounts.

BASIL (Sweet)

BOTANICAL NAME: *Ocimum basilicum*

FAMILY: Lamiaceae

The Plant: This bushy plant is native to Africa and Asia. Sweet basil grows to about 2 feet (60 cm) high and has white, blue, or purple flowers. There are over 150 varieties of basil.

The Essential Oil: The oil is extracted from the whole plant.

Scent of the Oil: Warm, spicy, licoricelike.

Main Uses

Purifying; calming; reduces stress; promotes restful sleep; mood uplifting; improves mental clarity, awareness, and memory; promotes dreaming; helps meditation; lessens pain; neutralizes toxins from insect bites.

Other Uses

Improves digestion; helps reduce cellulite; increases lactation; soothes insect bites.

Precautions: People with dry or sensitive skin may require additional carrier oil when using basil oil on the skin. Use small amounts.

BAY (West Indian)

BOTANICAL NAME: *Pimenta racemosa*

FAMILY: Myrtaceae

The Plant: This tropical evergreen tree is native to the West Indies. The tree grows to about 30 to 50 feet (9 to 15 m) high and has aromatic, leathery leaves and clusters of white or pink flowers that develop into black oval berries.

The Essential Oil: The oil is extracted from the leaves of the tree.

Scent of the Oil: Warm, sweet, spicy, balsamic.

Main Uses

Warming; improves circulation; purifying; improves mental clarity and alertness; relieves aching limbs and muscles; lessens pain; soothes sprains; disinfectant.

Other Uses

Vapors open sinuses and breathing passages; stimulates digestion; helps reduce cellulite; calming; reduces stress; promotes perspiration; repels insects.

Precautions: People with dry or sensitive skin may require additional carrier oil when using bay oil on the skin. Use small amounts.

BERGAMOT

BOTANICAL NAME: *Citrus bergamia*
FAMILY: Rutaceae

The Plant: The evergreen citrus tree is native to Asia and grows to about 15 feet (4.5 m) high. The tree bears a green to yellow fruit.

The Essential Oil: The oil is extracted from the peel of the fruit of the tree.

Scent of the Oil: Citruslike, sweet, slightly floral.

Main Uses

Purifying; balancing; calming; relieves anxiety, nervous tension, and stress; promotes restful sleep; mood uplifting; refreshing; improves mental clarity and alertness.

Other Uses

Cooling; helps reduce cellulite; disinfectant.

Precautions: People with dry or sensitive skin may require additional carrier oil when using bergamot oil on the skin. Avoid exposure to direct sunlight several hours after applying the oil.

BIRCH (Sweet)

BOTANICAL NAME: *Betula lenta*

FAMILY: Betulaceae

The Plant: Sweet birch, also known as black birch, is native to North America. The tree grows to about 50 to 80 feet (15 to 24 m) high and has black bark and leaves that smell like wintergreen.

The Essential Oil: The oil is extracted from the bark of the tree.

Scent of the Oil: Warm, root-beerlike.

Main Uses

Warming; improves circulation; purifying; relieves achy, tense, and sore muscles; reduces inflammation; lessens pain—especially in the joints.

Other Uses

Helps reduce cellulite; calming; relaxes nerves;

reduces tension and stress; promotes restful sleep; mood uplifting.

Comments: Sweet birch is rarely produced anymore, and it is commonly falsified with the synthetic chemical methyl salicylate.

Precautions: People with dry or sensitive skin may require additional carrier oil when using sweet birch oil on the skin. Use small amounts.

BLACK PEPPER

BOTANICAL NAME: *Piper nigrum*
FAMILY: Piperaceae
The Plant: Black pepper is a tropical climbing vine native to South India and Sri Lanka. The plant grows to about 10 feet (3 m) high and has spikes of small white flowers and clusters of small round fruits. As the berries ripen, they turn from green to orange to red. After the berries are picked, they are left to dry in the sun, which turns them black.
The Essential Oil: The oil is extracted from the fruits of the plant.
Scent of the Oil: Warm, peppery.

Main Uses

Warming; increases circulation; loosens tight muscles; improves the benefits of other oils when used together.

Other Uses

In small amounts improves digestion; reviving; stimulating; improves mental clarity.

Precautions: People with dry or sensitive skin may require additional carrier oil when using black pepper oil on the skin. Use small amounts.

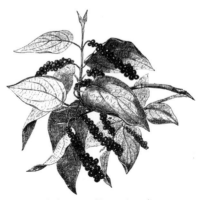

Black Pepper (*Piper nigrum*)

BOIS DE ROSE (Rosewood)

BOTANICAL NAME: *Aniba rosaeodora*

FAMILY: Lauraceae

The Plant: Bois de rose is an evergreen tree native to tropical American rainforests, the West Indies, and India. The tree grows to about 80 feet (24 m) high and has leathery leaves and red flowers.

The Essential Oil: The oil is extracted from the wood of the tree.

Scent of the Oil: Sweet, floral, woody.

Main Uses

Calming; relieves nervousness and stress; regenerates and moisturizes skin.

Other Uses

Mood uplifting; lessens pain.

CABREUVA

BOTANICAL NAME: *Myrocarpus fastigiatus*
FAMILY: Fabaceae
The Plant: Cabreuva is native to South America. The tree grows to about 50 feet (15 m) high in coastal forests.
The Essential Oil: The oil is extracted from the wood chips of the tree.
Scent of the Oil: Sweet, woody.

Main Uses

Warming; calming; reduces stress and tension; mood uplifting; improves mental clarity and alertness; loosens tight muscles; reduces pain.

Other Uses

Helpful for breathing; acts as euphoric and aphrodisiac.

CAJEPUT

BOTANICAL NAME: *Melaleuca cajuputi, M. leucadendron, M. minor*

FAMILY: Myrtaceae

The Plant: Cajeput is an evergreen tree native to Australia and Asia. The tree grows to about 50 to 100 feet (15 to 30 m) high and is cultivated as an ornamental tree for its white, pink, or purple flowers.

The Essential Oil: The oil is extracted from the leaves and twigs of the tree.

Scent of the Oil: Sweet, camphorous, vaporous.

Main Uses

Improves circulation; vapors open sinuses and breathing passages; relieves aches and pains.

Other Uses

Slightly warming; calming; reduces stress; promotes restful sleep; disinfectant; repels insects.

<u>CARAWAY</u>

BOTANICAL NAME: *Carum carvi*
FAMILY: Apiaceae
The Plant: Caraway is native to Europe and Asia. The plant grows to about 2 feet (60 cm) high, has carrotlike leaves and root, and small white or pink flowers which are followed by seed capsules that burst open when mature.
The Essential Oil: The oil is extracted from the seeds of the plant.
Scent of the Oil: Spicy.

Main Uses

Relieves pain; eases menstrual discomfort.

Other Uses

Improves digestion; soothes the intestines; relieves flatulence.

CARDAMOM

BOTANICAL NAME: *Elettaria cardamomum*
FAMILY: Zingiberaceae
The Plant: Cardamom is native to Asia. The plant grows to about 10 feet (3 m) high and has small yellow flowers. The fruit holds 18 seeds.
The Essential Oil: The oil is extracted from the seeds of the plant.
Scent of the Oil: Fresh, warm, spicy, vaporous.

Main Uses

Warming; improves circulation; mood uplifting; energizing; improves mental clarity; promotes physical strength; relieves pain; eases menstrual discomfort.

Other Uses

Improves digestion; soothes the intestines; relieves flatulence.

CASSIA BARK

BOTANICAL NAME: *Cinnamomum cassia*
FAMILY: Lauraceae
The Plant: Cassia is an evergreen tree native to Asia. The tree grows to about 40 to 80 feet (12 to 24 m) high and has a thin, peeling bark; long, glossy leathery leaves; and small green flowers that develop into berries, each of which contains a seed.
The Essential Oil: The oil is extracted from the bark of the tree.
Scent of the Oil: Warm, sweet, rich cinnamon.

Main Uses
Mood uplifting; reviving; improves mental clarity; disinfectant; insect repellant.

Precautions: Cassia bark oil is heating and can cause skin irritation. Avoid use on the skin.

CEDARWOOD (Atlas)

BOTANICAL NAME: *Cedrus atlantica*

FAMILY: Pinaceae

The Plant: Cedarwood is an evergreen tree native to Africa. The tree grows to about 130 to 140 feet (39 to 42 m) high and has needlelike leaves. Undisturbed trees can reach an age of 1,000 to 2,000 years old.

The Essential Oil: The oil is extracted from the wood of the tree.

Scent of the Oil: Sweet, floral, woody.

Main Uses

Improves mental clarity; promotes dreaming; aids meditation; loosens tight muscles; lessens pain.

Other Uses

Calming; relieves anxiety and nervous tension; promotes restful sleep; helpful for breathing; eases chest congestion when rubbed on the chest; mood uplifting; repels insects.

CELERY

Botanical Name: *Apium graveolens*
Family: Apiaceae
The Plant: Celery is native to the Mediterranean. The plant grows to about 1 to 2 feet (30 to 60 cm) high and has white flowers.
The Essential Oil: The oil is extracted from the seeds of the plant.
Scent of the Oil: Warm, spicy, celerylike.

Main Uses
Purifying; promotes calm, relaxed state and restful sleep.

Other Uses
Cooling; helps reduce cellulite.

Precautions: Celery oil tends to slow down reflexes. Avoid driving or doing anything that requires full attention after using the oil. Use small amounts.

CHAMOMILE
(German and Roman)

BOTANICAL NAME: (German) *Matricaria chamomilla, M. recutica;* (Roman) *Anthemis nobilis, Chamaemelum nobile*

FAMILY: Asteraceae

The Plant: Both German and Roman chamomile are native to Europe and Asia. German chamomile grows to about 3 feet (90 cm) high. Roman chamomile grows about 1 foot (30 cm) high. Both plants have daisylike flowers.

The Essential Oil: The oil is extracted from the flowers of the plant.

Scent of the Oil: German chamomile is fruity and applelike. Roman chamomile is sweet, applelike, and herbaceous.

Main Uses

Calming; promotes restful sleep; mood uplifting; lessens pain; eases menstrual discomfort; soothes inflammation; healing to the skin.

Other Uses

Improves digestion; soothes the intestines; acts as euphoric; soothes insect bites.

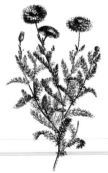

Roman Chamomile (*Anthemis nobilis*)

CHAMPACA FLOWER

BOTANICAL NAME: *Michelia alba, M. champaca*
FAMILY: Magnoliaceae
The Plant: Champaca is an evergreen tree native to Asia. The tree grows to about 65 feet (19.5 m) high and has long, glossy leaves and small, fragrant white flowers that develop into fruits with seeds inside.
The Essential Oil: The oil is extracted from the flowers of the tree.
Scent of the Oil: Sweet, floral.

Main Uses

Calming; reduces stress; promotes a peaceful state; mood uplifting.

Other Uses

Helpful for breathing; acts as euphoric.

<u>CINNAMON (Bark and Leaf)</u>

BOTANICAL NAME: *Cinnamomum verum, C. zeylanicum*
FAMILY: Lauraceae
The Plant: Cinnamon is an evergreen tree native to Asia. The tree grows to about 50 feet (15 m) high and has shiny green leathery leaves and clusters of small yellow flowers that develop into light blue berries.
The Essential Oil: The oil of cinnamon bark is extracted from the bark of the tree. The oil of cinnamon leaf is extracted from the leaves.
Scent of the Oil: Warm, sweet, cinnamon.

Main Uses

Heating; improves circulation; purifying; calming; relaxing; reduces stress; mood uplifting; reviving; helps relieve fatigue; improves mental clarity; loosens tight muscles; lessens pain; disinfectant.

Other Uses

Improves digestion; helps reduce cellulite; acts as euphoric; repels insects.

Precautions: People with dry or sensitive skin may require additional carrier oil when using cinnamon oil on the skin. Use small amounts.

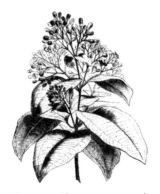

Cinnamon (*Cinnamomum verum*)

CLARY SAGE

BOTANICAL NAME: *Salvia sclarea*

FAMILY: Lamiaceae

The Plant: Clary sage is native to Europe. The plant grows to about 3 feet (90 cm) high and has whorls of pink, white, or blue flowers, depending on the variety.

The Essential Oil: The oil is extracted from the flowering tops of the plant.

Scent of the Oil: Sweet, herbaceous.

Main Uses

Calming; relieves stress and tension; promotes restful sleep; relieves pain; eases menstrual discomfort; regulates the female reproductive system.

Other Uses

Mood uplifting; aphrodisiac; improves digestion.

Precautions: Clary sage tends to slow down reflexes. Avoid driving or doing anything that requires full attention after using the oil. Use small amounts.

CLOVE BUD

BOTANICAL NAME: *Eugenia aromatica, Syzygium aromaticum*

FAMILY: Myrtaceae

The Plant: Clove is a tropical evergreen tree native to Asia. The tree grows to about 40 feet (12 m) high and has dark green leaves and bright pink buds that develop into yellow flowers, followed by purple berries.

The Essential Oil: The oil is extracted from the buds of the tree.

Scent of the Oil: Hot, spicy, sweet, penetrating.

Main Uses

Mood uplifting; reviving; mental stimulant; improves mental clarity and memory; disinfectant.

Other Uses

Warming; improves digestion; relieves flatulence; vapors open sinuses and breathing passages; aphrodisiac; reduces pain by numbing the area; repels insects.

Precautions: People with dry or sensitive skin may require additional carrier oil when using clove-bud oil on the skin. Use small amounts.

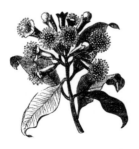

Clove (*Eugenia aromatica*)

COPAIBA

BOTANICAL NAME: *Copaifera officinalis*
FAMILY: Fabaceae
The Plant: Copaiba is an evergreen tree native to tropical America and Africa. The tree grows to about 60 feet (18 m) high and has small yellow flowers, followed by fruits that turn from brown to red.
The Essential Oil: The oil is extracted from the resin of the tree.
Scent of the Oil: Sweet, woody.

Main Uses

Calming; reduces stress; promotes a peaceful state of mind and restful sleep; opens breathing passages and allows deeper breathing; mood uplifting; improves mental clarity and alertness; helpful for meditation; healing and moisturizing to the skin; used as a fixative to hold the scent of a fragrance.

Other Uses

Soothes the intestines.

CORIANDER

BOTANICAL NAME: *Coriandrum sativum*
FAMILY: Apiaceae
The Plant: Coriander, also known as cilantro and Chinese parsley, is native to the Mediterranean. The plant grows to about 3 feet (90 cm) high and has small white flowers that develop into green seeds.
The Essential Oil: The oil is extracted from the seeds of the ripe fruits and the leaves of the plant.
Scent of the Oil: Warm, spicy, musky.

Main Uses
Reviving; energizing; helps relieve fatigue; improves mental clarity and memory; relieves pain.

Other Uses

Improves digestion; relieves flatulence, aerophagia, and nausea.

Precautions: Use small amounts.

CYPRESS

BOTANICAL NAME: *Cupressus sempervirens*
FAMILY: Cupressaceae

The Plant: Cypress is an evergreen tree native to Asia and the Mediterranean. The tree grows to about 80 to 160 feet (24 to 48 m) high and has dark green leaves and male and female cones that turn brown when mature. Some cypress trees are thought to be more than 3,000 years old.

The Essential Oil: The oil is extracted from the leaves and twigs of the tree.

Scent of the Oil: Turpentinelike, woody, penetrating.

Main Uses

Purifying; balances the nervous system; calming; relieves nervous tension and stress; promotes restful sleep; mood uplifting; refreshing; improves mental clarity and alertness; regulates the female reproductive and hormonal systems.

Other Uses
Helpful for breathing; helps reduce cellulite; contracts weak connective tissue; relieves muscle tension; lessens perspiration.

DILL

BOTANICAL NAME: *Anethum graveolens*
FAMILY: Apiaceae
The Plant: Dill is native to the Mediterranean and Russia. The plant grows to about 3 feet (90 cm) high and has feathery leaves and umbels of small yellow flowers that develop into aromatic seeds.
The Essential Oil: The oil is extracted from the whole plant or the seeds.
Scent of the Oil: Warm, spicy.

Main Uses

Calming; relaxing; promotes restful sleep; relieves pain; eases menstrual discomfort.

Other Uses

Improves digestion; soothes and freshens the intes--

tines; relieves flatulence and fermentation; repels insects.

Precautions: Dill tends to slow down reflexes. Avoid driving or doing anything that requires full attention after using the oil.

ELEMI

BOTANICAL NAME: *Canarium commune, C. luzonicum*
FAMILY: Burseraceae
The Plant: Elemi is an evergreen tree native to Asia. The tree grows to about 80 to 100 feet (24 to 30 m) high and has fragrant yellow flowers that develop into green fruits with nuts, called pili or Philippine nuts, which are an important food source. The tropical tree thrives in low elevations and a warm climate. A tree can bear up to 70 pounds (31.5 kg) of nuts annually.
The Essential Oil: The oil is extracted from the resin of the tree.
Scent of the Oil: Sweet, lemony, turpentinelike.

Main Uses

Calming; relaxing; reduces stress; promotes restful

sleep; helpful for meditation; encourages communication of inner feelings; healing to the skin.

Other Uses
Warming; improves circulation; opens breathing passages; breaks up mucus (mild effect); mood uplifting.

Precautions: Elemi tends to slow down reflexes. Avoid driving or doing anything that requires full attention after using the oil.

EUCALYPTUS & EUCALYPTUS RADIATA

BOTANICAL NAME: (Eucalyptus) *Eucalyptus globulus;* (Eucalyptus radiata) *Eucalyptus radiata*

FAMILY: Myrtaceae

The Plant: Eucalyptus globulus and eucalyptus radiata are evergreen trees native to Australia. The eucalyptus radiata tree grows to about 170 feet (51 m) high. Eucalyptus globulus, also known as gum tree, is one of the tallest of trees, reaching 300 to 480 feet (90 to 144 m) high. The leaves are fragrant and leathery. The flowers are white and the fruit is contained in a capsule.

The Essential Oil: The oil is extracted from the leaves of the tree.

Scent of the Oil: Fresh, camphorous, penetrating vapors.

Main Uses

Improves circulation; vapors open sinuses and breathing passages; mood uplifting; refreshing; reviving; energizing; improves mental clarity and alertness; relieves aching and sore muscles; lessens pain; disinfectant.

Other Uses

Cooling; repels insects.

Comments: Eucalyptus radiata is considered more gentle than eucalyptus globulus.

FENNEL (Sweet)

BOTANICAL NAME: *Foeniculum vulgare*
FAMILY: Apiaceae

The Plant: Fennel is native to Europe and Asia. The plant grows to about 3 to 7 feet (0.9 to 2.1 m) high and has dark green feathery leaves and clusters of small yellow flowers that develop into brownish gray seeds.

The Essential Oil: The oil is extracted from the seeds of the plant.

Scent of the Oil: Warm, fresh, sweet, licoricelike.

Main Uses

Warming; improves circulation; purifying; reduces stress; promotes restful sleep; relieves pain; eases menstrual discomfort.

Other Uses

Helpful for breathing; improves the digestion; soothes and purifies the intestines; relieves flatulence and aerophagia; helps reduce cellulite; increases lactation; disinfectant; repels insects.

Precautions: People with dry or sensitive skin may require additional carrier oil when using fennel oil on the skin. Sweet fennel tends to slow down reflexes. Avoid driving or doing anything that requires full attention after using the oil. Use small amounts. Avoid if prone to epileptic seizures.

FIR NEEDLES

BOTANICAL NAME: (Silver fir) *Abies alba;* (Grand fir) *Abies grandis;* (Fir balsam needle) *Abies balsamea;* (Douglas fir) *Pseudotsuga menziesii*

FAMILY: Pinaceae

The Plant: Fir is an evergreen tree native to North America and Europe. The trees can grow from 40 to 80 feet (12 to 24 m) or even 100 to 300 feet (30 to 90 m) high, depending on the species. The leaves are needlelike and the wood is soft and odorless. Fir trees are popular Christmas trees because the needles remain on the branches long after the tree has been cut.

The Essential Oil: The oil is extracted from the needles of the tree.

Scent of the Oil: Fresh, turpentinelike, sweet, balsamic.

Main Uses

Purifying; removes lymphatic deposits; calming; vapors open sinuses and breathing passages; mood uplifting; refreshing; reviving; improves mental clarity; encourages communication; lessens pain.

Other Uses

Helps reduce cellulite.

FRANKINCENSE

BOTANICAL NAME: *Boswellia carteri, B. thurifera*
FAMILY: Burseraceae
The Plant: Frankincense is native to the Mediterranean. The small tree grows to about 20 feet (6 m) high and has white flowers.
The Essential Oil: The oil is extracted from the gum that exudes from the bark of the tree.
Scent of the Oil: Fresh, balsamic, vaporous, with a lemony undertone.

Main Uses

Calming; relaxing; promotes restful sleep; vapors open sinuses and breathing passages; mood uplifting; brings out feelings; helpful for meditation; healing to the skin, especially bruises and burns; soothes inflamed skin.

GERANIUM

Botanical Name: *Pelargonium graveolens*
Family: Geraniaceae
The Plant: Geranium is a small fragrant plant native to Africa. The plant grows to about 3 feet (90 cm) high. There are over 700 species of geranium.
The Essential Oil: The oil is extracted from the leaves, stems, and flowers of the plant.
Scent of the Oil: Sweet, floral, musty.

Main Uses
Mood uplifting; improves mental clarity; encourages communication; purifying; lessens pain and inflammation.

Other Uses
Reduces tension; stimulates adrenal glands; reduces cellulite; disinfectant; repels insects and soothes bites.

GINGER

BOTANICAL NAME: *Zingiber officinale*
FAMILY: Zingiberaceae
The Plant: Ginger is native to Asia. The plant grows to about 3 feet (90 cm) high and has white or yellow flowers.
The Essential Oil: The oil is extracted from the rhizomes of the plant.
Scent of the Oil: Warm and spicy with a lemony undertone.

Main Uses

Warming; improves circulation; mood uplifting; improves mental clarity and the memory; general stimulant to the entire body; relieves dizziness and nausea caused by traveling; relieves aches and pains.

Other Uses

Improves digestion; soothes the intestines; relieves flatulence; cleanses the bowels; disinfectant.

Precautions: People with dry or sensitive skin may require additional carrier oil when using ginger oil on the skin. Use small amounts.

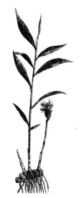

Ginger (*Zingiber officinale*)

GINGERGRASS

BOTANICAL NAME: *Cymbopogon martinii* var. *sofia*
FAMILY: Poaceae
The Plant: Gingergrass is a grass native to Asia. The plant, which is closely related to palmarosa, thrives in moist soils.
The Essential Oil: The oil is extracted from the grassy plant.
Scent of the Oil: Sharp, vaporous, warm, herbaceous, sweet.

Main Uses

Warming; improves circulation; calming; reduces stress; vapors open sinuses and breathing passages; reduces pain.

Other Uses

Mood uplifting; euphoric; aphrodisiac; improves mental clarity.

Precautions: People with dry or sensitive skin may require additional carrier oil when using gingergrass oil on the skin. Use small amounts.

GRAPEFRUIT

BOTANICAL NAME: *Citrus paradisi*
FAMILY: Rutaceae
The Plant: Grapefruit is an evergreen citrus tree that grows to about 30 to 50 feet (9 to 15 m) high and has glossy green leaves and fragrant white flowers that develop into large edible yellow fruits. Scientists believe that the tree may have developed as a mutation from the pomelo fruit.
The Essential Oil: The oil is extracted from the peel of the fruit of the tree.
Scent of the Oil: Light, fresh, citrus.

Main Uses

Purifying; reduces stress; mood uplifting; reviving; improves mental clarity and awareness.

Other Uses

Cooling; increases physical strength and energy; helps reduce cellulite; controls obesity; balances bodily fluids.

Precautions: People with dry or sensitive skin may require additional carrier oil when using grapefruit oil on the skin. Use small amounts. Avoid exposure to direct sunlight several hours after applying the oil.

GUAIACWOOD

BOTANICAL NAME: *Bulnesia sarmienti, Guaiacum officinale*
FAMILY: Zygophyllaceae

The Plant: Guaiacwood, also known as guaiacum, guayacan, pockwood, or lignum vitae ("wood of life"), is an evergreen tree native to the West Indies and Central America. The tree grows to about 40 feet (12 m) high and has leathery leaves and blue or purple flowers. The wood of the tree has a rich supply of fats and resins that make it very hard and impervious to water.

The Essential Oil: The resin or essential oil is extracted from the wood of the tree.

Scent of the Oil: Rich, sweet, fruity, woody.

Main Uses

Purifying; calming; relaxing; reduces stress and tension; promotes restful sleep; aids meditation; soothes swollen and injured skin tissue.

Other Uses
Mood uplifting; improves mental clarity; reduces inflammation; loosens tight muscles.

Precautions: Guaiacwood tends to slow down reflexes. Avoid driving or doing anything that requires full attention after using the oil.

HAVOZO BARK

BOTANICAL NAME: *Ravensara anisata*
FAMILY: Lauraceae
The Plant: Havozo is a small tree native to Madagascar.
The Essential Oil: The oil is extracted from the bark of the tree.
Scent of the Oil: Fresh, licoricelike, warm, sweet, vaporous.

Main Uses

Calming; reduces stress; promotes restful sleep; mood uplifting; encourages communication; relieves aches and pains; eases menstrual discomfort.

Other Uses

Warming; soothes intestines; vapors open sinuses

and breathing passages; euphoric; aphrodisiac; improves mental clarity; loosens tight muscles.

HELICHRYSUM

BOTANICAL NAME: *Helichrysum angustifolium, H. italicum*

FAMILY: Asteraceae

The Plant: Helichrysum, also known as everlasting or immortelle, is an evergreen plant native to the Mediterranean and Asia. The plant grows to about 2 feet (60 cm) high and has silvery green leaves and clusters of yellow flowers. There are over 500 species of helichrysum.

The Essential Oil: The oil is extracted from the flowers of the plant.

Scent of the Oil: Richly sweet, winelike.

Main Uses

Mood uplifting; reviving; strengthening; improves mental clarity and alertness; increases muscle endurance; relieves pain; eases menstrual discomfort.

Other Uses

Relaxing; reduces stress; vapors open sinuses and breathing passages; euphoric.

HYSSOP DECUMBENS

BOTANICAL NAME: *Hyssopus officinalis* var. *decumbens*

FAMILY: Lamiaceae

The Plant: Hyssop is a semievergreen plant native to Europe and Asia. The bushy plant grows to about 1 to 4 feet (30 to 120 cm) high and has aromatic leaves and spikes of white, pink, blue, or dark purple flowers.

The Essential Oil: The oil is extracted from the leaves and flowering tops of the plant.

Scent of the Oil: Sweet, camphorous, penetrating vapors.

Main Uses

Vapors open sinuses and breathing passages; mood uplifting; reviving; improves mental clarity and alertness.

Comments: Hyssop decumbens is more gentle than other varieties of hyssop.

Precautions: Avoid hyssop decumbens if prone to epileptic seizures.

JUNIPER BERRY

BOTANICAL NAME: *Juniperus communis*
FAMILY: Cupressaceae

The Plant: Juniper is an evergreen bush native to Europe, Asia, and Northern America. The bush grows to about 2 to 6 feet (60 cm to 1.8 m) high, sometimes reaching 25 feet (7.5 m) high. The male bushes have yellow cones and the female bushes have bluish green cones. The silvery green leaves are needlelike. The green berries take 3 years to ripen to a bluish black color. The bush can live to an age of 2,000 years.

The Essential Oil: The oil is extracted from the ripe berries of the bush.

Scent of the Oil: Fresh, clean, balsamic, turpentine-like, vaporous.

Main Uses

Purifying; relaxing; reduces stress; mood uplifting; refreshing; reviving; improves mental clarity and the memory; lessens pain; reduces swellings and fluid retention; eases menstrual discomfort.

Other Uses

Cleansing to the intestines and the tissues in the body; helps reduce cellulite; helpful for breathing; disinfectant; repels insects; soothes insect bites.

Precautions: Because of juniper berry's strong stimulating effect on the kidneys, use small amounts. Avoid use when the person has weak kidneys.

LABDANUM (Cistus)

BOTANICAL NAME: *Cistus ladanifer*

FAMILY: Cistaceae

The Plant: Labdanum, also called rockrose, is a small evergreen bush native to the Mediterranean and the Middle East. The bush grows to about 10 feet (3 m) high and has large white flowers.

The Essential Oil: The resin or essential oil is extracted from the leaves of the bush.

Scent of the Oil: Rich, winelike.

Main Uses

Calming; reduces stress; promotes restful sleep; mood uplifting; brings out feelings; encourages communication; helpful for meditation.

Other Uses
Warming; increases circulation; loosens tight muscles; euphoric; used as a fixative to hold the scent of a fragrance.

LAVENDER

BOTANICAL NAME: *Lavandula angustifolia, L. officinalis*
FAMILY: Lamiaceae
The Plant: Lavender is an evergreen plant native to the Mediterranean. The plant grows to about 3 feet (90 cm) high and has spikes of lilac-colored flowers. There are over 28 species of lavender.
The Essential Oil: The oil is extracted from the flowers of the plant.
Scent of the Oil: Fresh, herbaceous.

Main Uses

Calming; lessens tension; relaxes the muscles; promotes restful sleep; vapors open sinuses and breathing passages; purifying; lessens pains; healing to the skin, especially for bruises, cuts, wounds, burns, sunburns, scars, sores, insect bites, and injuries.

Other Uses

Improves digestion; soothing to the intestines; helps reduce cellulite; gently removes fluid retention; mood uplifting; balances mood swings; disinfectant; repels insects.

LEMON

BOTANICAL NAME: *Citrus limon*
FAMILY: Rutaceae
The Plant: Lemon is an evergreen citrus tree native to Asia. The tree grows to about 10 to 20 feet (3 to 6 m) high and has fragrant white flowers that develop into edible yellow fruits.
The Essential Oil: The oil is extracted from the peel of the fruit of the tree.
Scent of the Oil: Clean, fresh, lemon citrus.

Main Uses

Purifying; cleansing to the tissues; reduces cellulite and obesity; calming, relaxing; reduces stress; promotes restful sleep; mood uplifting; refreshing, reviving; improves mental clarity, alertness, and the memory; encourages communication.

Other Uses
Cooling; disinfectant; soothes insect bites.

Precautions: People with dry or sensitive skin may require additional carrier oil when using lemon oil on the skin. Use small amounts. Avoid exposure to direct sunlight for several hours after applying.

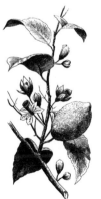

Lemon (*Citrus limon*)

LEMONGRASS

Botanical Name: *Cymbopogon citratus, C. flexuosus*
Family: Poaceae
The Plant: Lemongrass is native to Asia. The grass grows to about 2 feet (60 cm) high and has bulbous stems and swordlike leaves.
The Essential Oil: The oil is extracted from the whole plant, which is a grass.
Scent of the Oil: Rich, warm, strong lemon.

Main Uses

Balancing to the nervous system; calming; reduces stress; promotes restful sleep; mood uplifting; reviving; improves alertness.

Other Uses

Improves digestion; vapors open sinuses and breathing passages; reduces inflammation and swollen tissues; contracts weak connective tissue; tones skin; increases lactation; repels insects.

Precautions: People with dry or sensitive skin may require additional carrier oil when using lemongrass oil on the skin.

LIME

BOTANICAL NAME: *Citrus aurantiifolia, C. limetta*
FAMILY: Rutaceae
The Plant: Lime is an evergreen citrus tree native to Asia. The tree grows to about 10 feet (3 m) high and has fragrant white flowers that develop into edible green fruits.
The Essential Oil: The oil is extracted from the peel of the fruit of the tree.
Scent of the Oil: Rich, fresh, sweet, citrus.

Main Uses

Purifying; reduces stress; mood uplifting; refreshing; reviving; improves mental clarity and alertness; encourages communication.

Other Uses

Cooling; strengthens nerves; helpful when weakness in the body; helps reduce cellulite; disinfectant; soothes insect bites.

Precautions: People with dry or sensitive skin may require additional carrier oil when using lime oil on the skin. Use small amounts. Avoid exposure to direct sunlight several hours after applying the oil.

LITSEA CUBEBA

BOTANICAL NAME: *Litsea cubeba*
FAMILY: Lauraceae
The Plant: Litsea cubeba is an evergreen tree native to Asia. The tree grows to about 30 feet (9 m) high and has lemony scented leaves and white flowers that develop into small red or black berries.
The Essential Oil: The oil is extracted from the berries of the tree.
Scent of the Oil: Rich, heavy, lemon.

Main Uses

Calming; reduces stress; promotes restful sleep; mood uplifting; reviving; improves mental clarity and alertness.

Other Uses

Cooling; improves digestion; euphoric; relieves pain.

Precautions: People with dry or sensitive skin may require additional carrier oil when using litsea cubeba oil on the skin. Use small amounts.

MANDARIN

BOTANICAL NAME: *Citrus nobilis, C. reticulata*

FAMILY: Rutaceae

The Plant: Mandarin is an evergreen citrus tree native to Asia. The tree grows to about 20 to 25 feet (6 to 7.5 m) high and has glossy leaves and fragrant white flowers that develop into edible orange fruits.

The Essential Oil: The oil is extracted from the peel of the fruit of the tree.

Scent of the Oil: Fresh, sweet citrus, floral.

Main Uses

Calming; promotes restful sleep; mood uplifting; relieves emotional tension and stress; improves mental clarity and alertness; purifying.

Other Uses

Cooling; helps reduce cellulite.

Precautions: People with dry or sensitive skin may require additional carrier oil when using mandarin oil on the skin. Use small amounts. Avoid exposure to direct sunlight several hours after applying the oil.

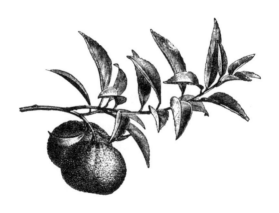

Mandarin Orange (*Citrus nobilis*)

MANUKA

BOTANICAL NAME: *Leptospermum scoparium*
FAMILY: Myrtaceae
The Plant: Manuka, also known as New Zealand tea tree or leptospermum, is an evergreen shrub native to New Zealand and Australia. The shrub grows to about 10 feet (3 m) high and has white, pink, or red flowers with a red center.
The Essential Oil: The oil is extracted from the leaves and branches of the shrub.
Scent of the Oil: Richly sweet.

Main Uses

Calming; reduces stress and tension; mood uplifting; improves mental clarity; loosens tight muscles; relieves pain; deodorant; healing to the skin.

Other Uses
Helpful for breathing; euphoric; aphrodisiac; disinfectant.

MARJORAM (Spanish and Sweet)

BOTANICAL NAME: (Spanish marjoram) *Thymus mastichina;* (sweet marjoram) *Majorana hortensis, Origanum majorana*

FAMILY: Lamiaceae

The Plant: Spanish marjoram is native to Spain. The plant grows to about 1 foot (30 cm) high and has small white flowers. Sweet marjoram is a bushy plant native to the Mediterranean. It grows to about 2 feet (60 cm) high and has light grayish green leaves and white or purple flowers.

The Essential Oil: The oil is extracted from the flowering tops and leaves of the plant.

Scent of the Oil: Warm, camphorous, vaporous, spicy.

Main Uses

Warming; improves circulation; relaxing; calms nervous tension; promotes restful sleep; vapors open sinuses and breathing passages; relaxes tense muscles; relieves pain; helps reduce inflammation and spasms; eases menstrual discomfort.

Other Uses

Improves digestion; disinfectant.

Precautions: Marjoram tends to slow down reflexes. Avoid driving or doing anything that requires full attention after using the oil. Use small amounts.

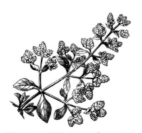

Marjoram (*Marjorana hortensis*)

<u>MYRRH</u>

BOTANICAL NAME: *Commiphora myrrha*
FAMILY: Burseraceae
The Plant: Myrrh is native to Africa and Asia. The tree grows to about 9 feet (2.7 m) high and has yellowish red flowers.
The Essential Oil: The resin or essential oil is extracted from the gum that exudes from the bark of the tree.
Scent of the Oil: Heavy, balsamic, smoky.

Main Uses

Calming; promotes restful sleep; helpful for meditation; healing to the skin.

Other Uses

Mood uplifting; soothes inflamed tissue; used as a fixative to hold the scent of a fragrance.

NEROLI

BOTANICAL NAME: *Citrus aurantium*
FAMILY: Rutaceae
The Plant: Bitter orange is an evergreen citrus tree native to Asia. The tree grows to about 20 to 30 feet (6 to 9 m) high and has fragrant white blossoms that yield neroli oil.
The Essential Oil: The oil is extracted from the blossoms of the tree.
Scent of the Oil: Sweet, floral, citrus.

Main Uses

Calms nervous tension; promotes restful sleep; mood uplifting; boosts confidence; helps in facing fears; eases menstrual discomfort.

Other Uses

Soothes the intestines; improves mental clarity.

NIAOULI

BOTANICAL NAME: *Melaleuca quinquenervia, M. viridiflora*

FAMILY: Myrtaceae

The Plant: Niaouli is an evergreen bush with yellow flowers that is native to Australia.

The Essential Oil: The oil is extracted from the leaves and twigs of the bush.

Scent of the Oil: Fresh, sweet, camphorous, penetrating vapors.

Main Uses

Vapors open sinuses and breathing passages; relieves aches and pain.

NUTMEG

BOTANICAL NAME: *Myristica fragrans*
FAMILY: Myristicaceae
The Plant: Nutmeg is an evergreen tree native to the Molucca Islands. The tree grows to about 60 to 80 feet (18 to 24 m) high and has pale yellow flowers that develop into fleshy yellow fruits that contain a single seed in a brown shell.
The Essential Oil: The oil is extracted from the seeds of the tree.
Scent of the Oil: Warm, spicy.

Main Uses
Calming; promotes restful sleep; promotes dreaming; loosens tight muscles.

Other Uses

Mood uplifting; relieves aches, pains, and sore muscles; eases menstrual discomfort.

Precautions: Nutmeg tends to slow down reflexes. Avoid driving or doing anything that requires full attention after using the oil. Use small amounts.

ORANGE

BOTANICAL NAME: (Bitter Orange) *Citrus aurantium*; (Sweet Orange) *Citrus sinensis*

FAMILY: Rutaceae

The Plant: Bitter orange and sweet orange are evergreen citrus trees native to Asia. The trees grow to about 20 to 30 feet (6 to 9 m) high and have fragrant white flowers that develop into edible orange-colored fruits.

The Essential Oil: The oil is extracted from the peel of the fruit of the tree.

Scent of the Oil: Fresh, sweet citrus.

Main Uses

Purifying; calming; reduces stress; promotes restful sleep; mood uplifting; relieves emotional tension and stress; improves mental clarity and alertness.

Other Uses

Cooling; helps reduce cellulite; relieves spasms.

Precautions: People with dry or sensitive skin may require additional carrier oil when using orange oil on the skin. Use small amounts. Avoid exposure to direct sunlight for several hours after applying the oil.

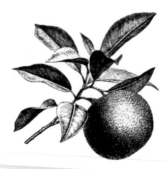

Sweet Orange (*Citrus sinensis*)

OREGANO

BOTANICAL NAME: *Origanum vulgare*
FAMILY: Lamiaceae
The Plant: Oregano is native to Europe and America. The plant grows to about 1 to 2 feet (30 to 60 cm) high and has dark green leaves and purple buds that blossom into white, pink, or lilac flowers. The entire plant is aromatic.
The Essential Oil: The oil is extracted from the flowering plant.
Scent of the Oil: Hot, spicy.

Main Uses

Heating; improves circulation; calming; relaxing; promotes restful sleep; relieves muscle pain; loosens tight muscles; increases physical strength and endurance.

Other Uses

Improves digestion; purifying; helps reduce cellulite; vapors open sinuses and breathing passages; mood uplifting; improves mental clarity and alertness; increases perspiration; disinfectant; repels insects.

Precautions: People with dry or sensitive skin may require additional carrier oil when using oregano oil on the skin. Use small amounts.

PALMAROSA

BOTANICAL NAME: *Cymbopogon martinii* var. *motia*
FAMILY: Poaceae
The Plant: Palmarosa is a fragrant grass native to Asia. The plant grows to about 9 feet (2.7 m) high and has clusters of flowers that turn red when mature.
The Essential Oil: The oil is extracted from the plant.
Scent of the Oil: Sweet and floral with a lemony undertone.

Main Uses

Calming; reduces stress; reduces pain and inflammation; moisturizing and regenerating to the skin.

Other Uses

Warming; improves circulation; mood uplifting; refreshing; improves mental clarity.

<u>PATCHOULI</u>

BOTANICAL NAME: *Pogostemon patchouli*
FAMILY: Lamiaceae
The Plant: Patchouli is native to Asia. The plant grows to about 3 feet (90 cm) high and has whorls of light purple or lavender flowers. Patchouli requires full sun to bring out its fragrance.
The Essential Oil: The oil is extracted from the leaves of the plant.
Scent of the Oil: Heavy, earthy.

Main Uses

Mood uplifting; aphrodisiac; used as a fixative to hold the scent of a fragrance.

Other Uses

Stimulating; prevents sleep; euphoric; healing to the skin; repels insects.

PEPPERMINT

BOTANICAL NAME: *Mentha piperita*
FAMILY: Lamiaceae

The Plant: Peppermint is a cross between several wild mints. The true peppermint plant cannot reproduce and is propagated through the root system below the soil. The plant grows to about 1 to 3 feet (30 to 90 cm) high and has a purplish stem and pale violet flowers.

The Essential Oil: The oil is extracted from the flowering tops of the plant.

Scent of the Oil: Fresh, sweet mint, penetrating vapors.

Main Uses

Vapors open sinuses and breathing passages; mood uplifting; refreshing; reviving; stimulating; improves mental clarity, alertness, memory, and ability to concentrate; encourages communication; increases physical strength and endurance; relieves pain and inflammation; eases menstrual discomfort.

Other Uses

Cooling; improves digestion; increases appetite; relieves flatulence and nausea; sweetens the intestines; freshens bad breath; euphoric; aphrodisiac; reduces lactation; repels insects; kills parasites; soothes itching skin.

Precautions: People with dry or sensitive skin may require additional carrier oil when using peppermint oil on the skin. Use small amounts.

PETITGRAIN

BOTANICAL NAME: (Bitter Orange) *Citrus bigaradia*
FAMILY: Rutaceae
The Plant: Petitgrain oil is obtained from the leaves and twigs of the evergreen citrus trees orange, lemon, or tangerine, all of which are native to Asia.
The Essential Oil: The oil is extracted from the leaves and twigs of the tree.
Scent of the Oil: Citrus, herbaceous.

Main Uses

Calms the nerves; relieves anxiety, tension, and mental stress; promotes restful sleep; mood uplifting; improves mental clarity and alertness; helpful for meditation.

Other Uses

Cooling; soothes inflamed and irritated skin tissue.

PIMENTO BERRY (Allspice)

BOTANICAL NAME: *Pimenta dioica, P. officinalis*
FAMILY: Myrtaceae
The Plant: Allspice is an evergreen tree native to the West Indies and Central America. The tree grows to about 30 to 70 feet (9 to 21 m) high and has leathery leaves and small white flowers that develop into aromatic berries that turn dark brown when ripe.
The Essential Oil: The oil is extracted from the dried unripe berries of the tree.
Scent of the Oil: Warm, spicy, sweet, cinnamon-clovelike.

Main Uses

Warming; improves circulation; purifying; calms the nerves; removes stress; promotes restful sleep; mood uplifting; loosens tight muscles; lessens pain.

Other Uses

Vapors open sinuses and breathing passages; improves digestion; helps reduce cellulite.

Precautions: People with dry or sensitive skin may require additional carrier oil when using pimento-berry oil on the skin.

PINE

BOTANICAL NAME: *Pinus sylvestris*
FAMILY: Pinaceae
The Plant: Pine is an evergreen tree native to Asia and Europe. The tree grows to about 115 to 130 feet (34.5 to 39 m) high and has greenish blue needlelike leaves. A pine tree can live to an age of 1,200 years.
The Essential Oil: The oil is extracted from the needles and small branches of the tree.
Scent of the Oil: Fresh, turpentinelike, penetrating vapors.

Main Uses

Purifying; removes lymphatic deposits from the body; vapors open sinuses and breathing passages; mood uplifting; refreshing; reviving; improves mental clarity, alertness, and memory.

Other Uses

Helps reduce cellulite; stimulates the adrenal glands; promotes vitality; lessens pain; disinfectant.

Precautions: Pine oil has a strong diuretic effect on the kidneys and can also irritate the skin. Use small amounts with care.

RAVENSARA AROMATICA

BOTANICAL NAME: *Ravensara aromatica*

FAMILY: Lauraceae

The Plant: Ravensara aromatica is a small tree with fragrant flowers, leaves, and bark, native to Madagascar.

The Essential Oil: The oil is extracted from the leaves of the tree.

Scent of the Oil: Camphorous, penetrating vapors.

Main Uses

Vapors open sinuses and breathing passages; mood uplifting; refreshing; improves mental clarity; relieves pain.

Other Uses

Calming; reduces stress.

ROSE

BOTANICAL NAME: *Rosa centifolia, R. damascena*
FAMILY: Rosaceae
The Plant: Rose is native to the Mediterranean. There are many varieties of the rose bush that grow to various heights and produce sweet, fragrant flowers.
The Essential Oil: The oil is extracted from the flowers of the bush.
Scent of the Oil: Sweet, floral.

Main Uses

Purifying; mood uplifting; aphrodisiac; calms emotional shock and grief; balances the female hormonal and reproductive system; regenerates skin cells.

Other Uses

Calming; reduces stress; lessens pain and inflammation.

ROSEMARY

BOTANICAL NAME: *Rosmarinus officinalis*
FAMILY: Lamiaceae
The Plant: Rosemary is an evergreen shrub native to the Mediterranean. The bushy plant grows to about 2 to 6 feet (60 cm to 1.8 m) high and has needle-shaped leaves and small blue flowers. The entire plant is aromatic.
The Essential Oil: The oil is extracted from the flowers and leaves of the shrub.
Scent of the Oil: Camphorous, penetrating vapors.

Main Uses
Warming; improves circulation; purifying; removes lymphatic desposits from the body; vapors open sinuses and breathing passages; mood uplifting; refreshing; stimulating; improves mental clarity, alertness, and the memory; lessens pain.

Other Uses

Improves the digestion; helps reduce cellulite; disinfectant; repels insects.

Precautions: Avoid use rosemary if prone to epileptic seizures.

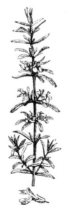

Rosemary (*Rosmarinus officinalis*)

SAGE (Spanish)

BOTANICAL NAME: *Salvia lavandulifolia*

FAMILY: Lamiaceae

The Plant: Spanish sage is an evergreen plant native to Spain. The plant grows to about 2fi feet (75 cm) high and has small purple flowers.

The Essential Oil: The oil is extracted from the flowers and leaves of the plant.

Scent of the Oil: Camphorous, penetrating vapors.

Main Uses

Improves circulation; purifying; reduces stress; improves alertness; lessens pain; eases menstrual discomfort.

Other Uses

Improves digestion; helps reduce cellulite; relaxes sore muscles; strengthens the body; suppresses perspiration and lactation.

Comments: Spanish sage is more gentle than common sage.

Precautions: Use small amounts. Avoid the oil if prone to epileptic seizures.

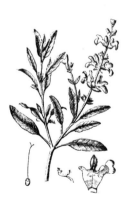

Sage (*Salvia lavandulifolia*)

SANDALWOOD

BOTANICAL NAME: *Santalum album*
FAMILY: Santalaceae
The Plant: Sandalwood is an evergreen tree native to Asia. The tree grows to about 30 feet (9 m) high and has small purple flowers and small fruits that contain a seed.
The Essential Oil: The oil is extracted from the inner wood of the tree.
Scent of the Oil: Sweet, woody.

Main Uses

Calming; relaxing, reduces stress; promotes restful sleep; encourages dreaming; helpful for meditation; mood uplifting; aphrodisiac; brings out emotions; healing and moisturizing to the skin; used as a fixative to hold the scent of a fragrance.

Other Uses
Soothing to the breathing passages; euphoric.

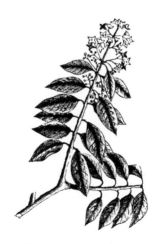

Sandalwood (*Santalum album*)

SPEARMINT

BOTANICAL NAME: *Mentha spicata, M. viridis*
FAMILY: Lamiaceae
The Plant: Spearmint is native to the Mediterranean. The plant grows to about 1 to 3 feet (30 to 90 cm) high and has shiny green leaves and white or lilac flowers.
The Essential Oil: The oil is extracted from the leaves and flowering tops of the plant.
Scent of the Oil: Fresh, sweet mint, penetrating vapors.

Main Uses

Vapors open sinuses and breathing passages; mood uplifting; refreshing; reviving; stimulating; aphrodisiac; improves mental clarity, alertness, ability to concentrate, and memory; encourages communication; increases physical strength and endurance; relieves pain and inflammation; eases menstrual discomfort.

Other Uses

Cooling; improves digestion; increases the appetite; relieves flatulence; freshens the breath and the intestines; repels insects; soothes itching skin.

Precautions: People with dry or sensitive skin may require additional carrier oil when using spearmint oil on the skin.

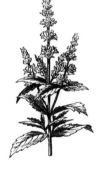

Spearmint (*Mentha viridis*)

SPIKENARD

BOTANICAL NAME: *Nardostachys jatamansi*
FAMILY: Valerianaceae
Also known as musk root.

The Plant: Spikenard is native to the Himalaya Mountains and Asia. The aromatic plant grows to about 2 feet (60 cm) high and has pink bell-shaped flowers.

The Essential Oil: The oil is extracted from the roots of the plant.

Scent of the Oil: Sweet, earthy.

Main Uses
Calming; relaxing; reduces stress; promotes restful sleep; mood uplifting; reduces inflammation.

SPRUCE

BOTANICAL NAME: *Picea mariana*
FAMILY: Pinaceae

The Plant: Spruce is an evergreen tree native to North America. The tree grows to about 70 to 200 feet (21 to 60 m) high and has bluish green needle-like leaves, purple flowers, and purple male and female cones that mature to a brownish color. The trees can live to an age of 1,200 years.

The Essential Oil: The oil is extracted from the needles of the tree.

Scent of the Oil: Fresh, sweet, turpentinelike, vaporous.

Main Uses

Calming; reduces stress; vapors open sinuses and breathing passages; mood uplifting; improves mental clarity; brings out inner feelings; encourages communication.

Other Uses

Euphoric; disinfectant.

ST.-JOHN'S-WORT

BOTANICAL NAME: *Hypericum perforatum*
FAMILY: Guttiferae
The Plant: St.-John's-wort is native to Europe, Asia, and Africa. The plant grows to about 1 to 3 feet (30 to 90 cm) high with star-shaped yellow flowers. When pinched, the flower petals turn red.
The Essential Oil: The oil is extracted from the blossoms of the plant.
Scent of the Oil: Sweet, floral.

Main Uses

Calming; reduces stress; mood uplifting; improves mental clarity; relieves pain; eases menstrual discomfort.

Other Uses

Euphoric; soothes the intestines.

Precautions: Avoid exposure to direct sunlight several hours after applying the oil on the skin.

TANGERINE

BOTANICAL NAME: *Citrus reticulata*

FAMILY: Rutaceae

The Plant: Tangerine is an evergreen citrus tree native to Asia. The tree grows to about 20 to 25 feet (6 to 7.5 m) high and has fragrant white flowers that develop into edible orange-colored fruits.

The Essential Oil: The oil is extracted from the peel of the fruit of the tree.

Scent of the Oil: Sweet, citrus.

Main Uses

Purifying; calming; relieves emotional tension and stress; promotes restful sleep; mood uplifting; improves mental clarity and alertness.

Other Uses

Cooling; helps reduce cellulite.

Precautions: People with dry or sensitive skin may require additional carrier oil when using tangerine oil on the skin. Avoid exposure to direct sunlight several hours after applying the oil.

<u>TEA TREE</u>

BOTANICAL NAME: *Melaleuca alternifolia*
FAMILY: Myrtaceae
The Plant: Tea tree is an evergreen tree native to Australia. The tree grows to about 10 feet (3 m) high and has needlelike leaves and purple or yellow flowers.
The Essential Oil: The oil is extracted from the leaves and twigs of the tree.
Scent of the Oil: Musty, camphorous, vaporous.

Main Uses

Relieves pain; disinfectant; healing to the skin, soothes insect bites.

Other Uses

Vapors open sinuses and breathing passages; mood uplifting; reviving; improves mental clarity.

<u>THYME</u>

BOTANICAL NAME: *Thymus aestivus, T. ilerdensis, T. valentinus, T. webbianus;* (Sweet Thyme) *Thymus satureiodes, T. vulgaris* var. *linalol*

FAMILY: Lamiaceae

The Plant: Thyme is an evergreen plant native to the Mediterranean. The plant grows about 1 foot (30 cm) high and has small gray-green leaves and white, pink, or pale lilac flowers.

The Essential Oil: The oil is extracted from the leaves and flowering tops of the plant.

Scent of the Oil: Warm, sharp, spicy, herbaceous.

Main Uses

Heating; improves circulation; purifying; vapors open sinuses and breathing passages; mood uplifting; stimulating; improves mental clarity and alertness; increases physical strength and energy; relieves pain, inflammation, and spasms; disinfectant.

Other Uses
Relaxes the nerves; improves digestion; cleanses the intestines; helps eliminate cellulite, waste material, and excessive fluids from the body; induces perspiration; repels insects; kills lice.

Comments: Thymus satureiodes and *Thymus vulgaris* var. *linalol* are less irritating to the skin and more gentle than common thyme.

Precautions: People with dry or sensitive skin may require additional carrier oil when using thyme oil on the skin. Use small amounts. Avoid thyme if you are prone to epileptic seizures.

VANILLA

BOTANICAL NAME: *Vanilla fragrans, V. planifolia*
FAMILY: Orchidaceae
The Plant: Vanilla is native to Mexico and Central America. The climbing plant reaches to about 12 feet (3.6 m) high and has clusters of pale yellow-green flowers followed by green pods containing many small seeds.
The Essential Oil: The oil is extracted from the unripe pods of the plant.
Scent of the Oil: Richly sweet, smoky.

Main Uses

Calming; reduces stress; promotes restful sleep; encourages dreaming; mood uplifting; aphrodisiac.

Other Uses

Euphoric.

Comments: For the formulas given in this book, it is recommended that the vanilla CO_2 extracted oil be used. The oil separates; therefore, the bottle may need to be placed in a warm container of water to make the consistency more uniform.

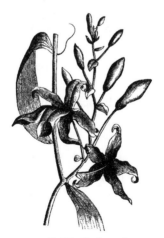

Vanilla (*Vanilla fragrans*)

VETIVER

BOTANICAL NAME: *Vetiveria zizanoides*
FAMILY: Poaceae

The Plant: Vetiver is native to Asia. The tropical grass grows to about 4 to 8 feet (1.2 to 2.4 m) high. Since its strong roots reach deep below the soil, the plant can help protect steep hillsides and areas vulnerable to soil erosion.

The Essential Oil: The oil is extracted from the roots of the grass.

Scent of the Oil: Rich, heavy, earthy.

Main Uses

Calms nervousness; relieves stress and tension; promotes restful sleep; strengthens the body; loosens tight muscles; relieves pain; healing to the skin; used as a fixative to hold the scent of a fragrance.

Other Uses

Improves digestion; mood uplifting; repels insects.

Comments: Vetiver oil is a thick oil and may need to be thinned in order to remove it from the bottle with a dropper. Therefore, place the bottle in a warm container of water before using.

YLANG-YLANG

BOTANICAL NAME: *Cananga odorata* var. *genuina*
FAMILY: Annonaceae
The Plant: Ylang-ylang is an evergreen tree native to
Asia. The tree grows to about 100 feet (30 m) high and
has glossy leaves and large yellow fragrant flowers.
The Essential Oil: The oil is extracted from the flow-
ers of the tree.
Scent of the Oil: Heavy, sweet, floral.

Main Uses

Calming; relaxing; reduces stress; promotes restful
sleep; mood uplifting; aphrodisiac; brings out feelings; enhances communication; loosens tight
muscles; lessens pain.

Other Uses

Euphoric; disinfectant.

CHAPTER 9

Carrier Oil Profiles

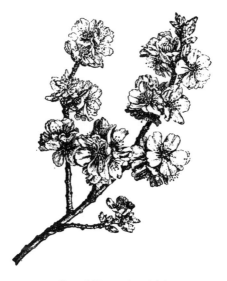

Almond (*Prunus Amygdalus*)

The role of carrier oils in aromatherapy is to dilute essential oils for use in massage, skin, and hair care blends. These oils moisturize, soothe, soften, nourish, and protect skin as they are absorbed deep into skin layers. Whenever essential oils are applied topically, carrier oils are combined with them to form a blend.

ALMOND (Sweet)

BOTANICAL NAME: *Prunus amygdalus, P. dulcis*
FAMILY: Rosaceae

The Plant: Sweet almond is native to Asia and the Mediterranean. The medium-size tree grows to about 35 feet (10.5 m) high and has pinkish white flowers followed by green fruits, each containing a nut.

The Carrier Oil: The oil is obtained from the nut of the tree.

Practical Uses
Skin and hair care; moisturizing.

APRICOT KERNEL

BOTANICAL NAME: *Armeniaca vulgaris, Prunus armeniaca*

FAMILY: Rosaceae

The Plant: Apricot is native to Asia. The tree grows to about 35 feet (10.5 m) high and has white to pink flowers followed by orange-yellow fruit.

The Carrier Oil: The oil is obtained from the kernel of the fruit.

Practical Uses

Skin care; moisturizing.

Apricot (*Armeniaca vulgaris*)

AVOCADO

BOTANICAL NAME: *Persea americana, P. gratissima*
FAMILY: Lauraceae
The Plant: Avocado is an evergreen tree native to the Americas. The tree grows to about 30 to 60 feet (9 to 18 m) high and has dark green oval leaves and greenish yellow flowers that develop into yellow, green, red, or purple fruit. The pulp is soft and buttery with a large pit inside. Avocado grows in many tropical regions.
The Carrier Oil: The oil is obtained from the kernel and fruit of the tree.

Practical Uses

Skin and hair care; moisturizing; purifies the skin. For massage blends, mix about 20 percent avocado oil with another carrier oil before adding the essential oils.

Comments: Avocado oil is very nourishing to the skin and contains vitamins A and E and especially large amounts of vitamin D and potassium. The avocado has the highest protein content of any fruit. The oil is extensively used in cosmetics.

BORAGE

BOTANICAL NAME: *Borago officinalis*
FAMILY: Boraginaceae
The Plant: Borage is native to the Mediterranean. The plant grows to about 2 to 4 feet (0.6 to 1.2 m) high and has large pointed oval leaves, hairy stems, and star-shaped, sky-blue flowers with a dark stamen in the center. The scent of the plant is similar to that of a cucumber.
The Carrier Oil: The oil is obtained from the seeds of the plant.

Practical Uses

Calming; eases PMS and menstrual discomfort; reduces inflammation; skin and hair care; moisturizes; soothes inflamed skin. For massage blends, mix about 20 percent borage oil with another carrier oil before adding essential oils.

CALOPHYLLUM

BOTANICAL NAME: *Calophyllum inophyllum*
FAMILY: Guttiferae
The Plant: Calophyllum is an evergreen tree commonly found in tropical Asia. The tree grows to about 100 feet (30 m) high and has white flowers that emit a sweet fragrance. The flowers develop into fruits that have a thin pulp and taste similar to apples.
The Carrier Oil: The oil is obtained from the kernel of the fruit.

Practical Uses

Skin and hair care; soothing to the skin. For massage blends, mix about 50 percent calophyllum oil with another carrier oil before adding essential oils.

CAMELLIA

BOTANICAL NAME: *Camellia japonica*
FAMILY: Theaceae
The Plant: Camellia grows wild in the mountains of Japan and China. The plant grows to about 6 to 20 feet (1.8 to 6 m) high and has showy flowers that develop into seeds. Camellia is a relative of trees that produce tea leaves. The plant thrives in cold climates of Asia, blossoming in winter, even in snow.
The Carrier Oil: The oil is obtained from the seeds of the plant.

Practical Uses

Skin and hair care; soothing to the skin.

COCOA BUTTER

BOTANICAL NAME: *Theobroma cacao*

FAMILY: Sterculiaceae

The Plant: Cocoa is an evergreen tree native to Central America. The tree grows to about 24 feet (7.2 m) high and has large, glossy leaves and small yellow flowers that develop into yellow or red fruits that contain many beanlike seeds.

The Carrier Oil: The butter is obtained from the beans of the tree.

Practical Uses

Stimulant to the body; skin and hair care; moisturizing.

EVENING PRIMROSE

BOTANICAL NAME: *Oenothera biennis*
FAMILY: Onagraceae

The Plant: Evening primrose is a plant that grows to about 1 to 8 feet (30 cm to 2.4 m) high and has long, pointed leaves and many fragrant yellow flowers that open at dusk to attract night-flying insects for pollination. Following the flowers are capsules that contain many small brownish-colored seeds. The plant originated in North America and was exported to Europe during the seventeenth century.

The Carrier Oil: The oil is obtained from the seeds of the plant.

Practical Uses

Reduces PMS and eases menstrual discomfort; reduces inflammation. Skin care; moisturizing;

soothing to the skin. For massage blends, mix about 20 percent evening primrose oil with another carrier oil before adding essential oils.

FLAXSEED

BOTANICAL NAME: *Linum usitatissimum*
FAMILY: Linaceae
The Plant: Although flax has been cultivated since ancient times, its origins are uncertain. The plant grows to about 2 feet (60 cm) high and has sky-blue flowers followed by brown seeds.
The Carrier Oil: The oil is obtained from the seeds of the plant.

Practical Uses
Skin care.

GRAPESEED

BOTANICAL NAME: *Vitis vinifera*

FAMILY: Vitaceae

The Plant: The grape plant is a climbing vine native to Asia. The vine grows to about 30 feet (9 m) high and has green flowers that develop into bunches of sweet-flavored green or purple fruits.

The Carrier Oil: The oil is obtained from the seeds of the fruit.

Practical Uses

Skin and hair care.

HAZELNUT

BOTANICAL NAME: *Corylus avellana*
FAMILY: Betulaceae
The Plant: Hazelnut, also called filbert and cobnut, is a deciduous tree native to Europe and Asia. The tree grows to about 12 to 30 feet (3.6 to 9 m) high and has budlike female flowers, yellowish brown male catkins, and clusters of nuts.
The Carrier Oil: The oil is obtained from the nut of the tree.

Practical Uses
Skin and hair care; moisturizing; softens and repairs dry or damaged skin.

JOJOBA

BOTANICAL NAME: *Simmondsia chinensis*
FAMILY: Buxaceae
The Plant: Jojoba is an evergreen shrub native to the southwestern United States and northern Mexico. The plant grows to about 3 to 18 feet (0.9 to 5.4 m) high and has small leathery leaves. The male plant has yellow flowers, and the female plant has green flowers that develop into olive-shaped fruits containing seeds inside. These seeds are called goat nut. Jojoba plants may live up to 200 years.
The Carrier Oil: The vegetable wax or oil is obtained from the beans of the shrub.

Practical Uses

Skin and hair care; moisturizing; minimizes stretch marks; used to protect the skin from the sun. For massage blends, mix about 50 percent jojoba oil with another carrier oil before adding essential oils.

Comments: Jojoba oil is stable and, if stored properly, has a very long shelf life.

KUKUI NUT

BOTANICAL NAME: *Aleurites moluccana*

FAMILY: Euphorbiaceae

The Plant: Kukui is an evergreen tree, native to Asia. The tree grows to about 70 feet (21 m) high and has white flowers that develop into fruits that contains a nut inside. Kukui is the state tree of Hawaii. It is also called varnish, candlenut, and candleberry tree.

The Carrier Oil: The oil is obtained from the nut of the tree.

Practical Uses

Skin and hair care; balancing, rejuvenating, and softening to the skin.

MACADAMIA NUT

BOTANICAL NAME: *Macadamia integrifolia*
FAMILY: Protoceae
The Plant: Macadamia is an evergreen tree native to Australia. The tree grows to about 30 to 70 feet (9 to 21 m) high and has shiny leaves and white flowers that develop into nuts. Macadamia was domesticated in Australia in the mid-nineteenth century.
The Carrier Oil: The carrier oil is obtained from the nut of the tree.

Practical Uses
Skin and hair care; softens and restores the skin.

ROSE HIP SEED

BOTANICAL NAME: *Rosa rubiginosa*

FAMILY: Rosaceae

The Plant: Rose is native to the Mediterranean. There are many varieties of the rosebush that grow to various heights and produce fragrant flowers in a wide range of colors.

The Carrier Oil: The carrier oil is obtained from the hips and seeds of the bush.

Practical Uses

Skin care; moisturizing; regenerating to the skin; reduces wrinkles.

SESAME

BOTANICAL NAME: *Sesamum indicum*
FAMILY: Pedaliaceae
The Plant: Sesame is native to Africa and Asia. The plant grows to about 3 to 6 feet (0.9 to 1.8 m) high and has oval leaves and white or pink tubular flowers with purple spots. The seeds can be white, yellow, red, brown, or black.
The Carrier Oil: The oil is obtained from the seeds of the plant. Sesame oil is also known as benne oil, gingle oil, and teel oil.

Practical Uses

Skin and hair care; moisturizing; soothing to the skin.

SHEA BUTTER

BOTANICAL NAME: *Butyrosperum parkii*
FAMILY: Sapotaceae
The Plant: Shea is native to Africa. The tree grows to about 70 feet (21 m) high and has white flowers with a sweet fragrance. The fruit is brown with a large white kernel inside.
The Butter: The butter is obtained from the nut kernels of the tree.

Practical Uses

Skin and hair care; moisturizing; suntan crème; massage crème.

MEASUREMENTS & EQUIVALENTS
∿

CAPACITY, Liquid or Dry Measure

⅕ teaspoon = 1 milliliter = 20 drops

1 teaspoon = 5 milliliters = 100 drops

1 tablespoon = 3 teaspoons = 15 milliliters = 300 drops

2 tablespoons = 1 fluid ounce = 30 milliliters = 600 drops

16 tablespoons = 1 cup = 8 fluid ounces = 240 milliliters

WEIGHT

1 ounce = 28.35 grams (rounded off to 28 grams)

3½ ounces = 99.26 grams (rounded off to 100 grams)

16 ounces = 1 pound = 454 grams

ABBREVIATIONS

t = teaspoon(s)   T = tablespoon(s)

fl oz = fluid ounce(s)   ml = milliliter(s)   L = liter(s)

oz = ounce(s)   g = gram(s)

cm = centimeter(s)   m = meter(s)

WEIGHTS OF COMMON INGREDIENTS

Arrowroot Powder 4 tablespoons (60 ml) weighs about 1½ ounces or 42 grams.

Bicarbonate of Soda ½ cup or 8 tablespoons (120 ml) weighs about 5 ounces or 142 grams.

Cocoa Butter 7 teaspoons (35 ml) weighs about 24.5 grams, a little less than 1 ounce.

Cornstarch 4 tablespoons (60 ml) weighs about 1 ounce or 28 grams.

Epsom Salts 1 cup (240 ml) weighs about 10 ounces or 284 grams.

Sea Salt 1 cup (240 ml) weighs about 10 ounces or 284 grams.

Shea Butter 2 tablespoons (30 ml) weighs about 1 ounce or 28 grams.

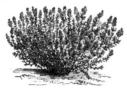

Thyme (*Thymus satureiodes*)

Index

If you liked this book, you'll love this series:

Little Giant Book of Optical Illusions • Little Giant Book of "True" Ghost Stories • Little Giant Book of Whodunits • Little Giant Encyclopedia of Aromatherapy • Little Giant Encyclopedia of Baseball Quizzes • Little Giant Encyclopedia of Card & Magic Tricks • Little Giant Encyclopedia of Card Games • Little Giant Encyclopedia of Card Games Gift Set • Little Giant Encyclopedia of Dream Symbols • Little Giant Encyclopedia of Fortune Telling • Little Giant Encyclopedia of Gambling Games • Little Giant Encyclopedia of Games for One or Two • Little Giant Encyclopedia of Handwriting Analysis • Little Giant Encyclopedia of Magic • Little Giant Encyclopedia of Mazes • Little Giant Encyclopedia of Names • Little Giant Encyclopedia of Natural Healing • Little Giant Encyclopedia of One-Liners • Little Giant Encyclopedia of Palmistry • Little Giant Encyclopedia of Puzzles • Little Giant Encyclopedia of Spells & Magic • Little Giant Encyclopedia of Superstitions • Little Giant Encyclopedia of Toasts & Quotes • Little Giant Encyclopedia of Travel & Holiday Games • Little Giant Encyclopedia of Word Puzzles • Little Giant Encyclopedia of the Zodiac

Available at fine stores everywhere.